Writing Works

Writing Works

A Resource Handbook for Therapeutic Writing Workshops and Activities

*Edited by Gillie Bolton, Victoria Field
and Kate Thompson*

Foreword by Blake Morrison

Jessica Kingsley Publishers
London and Philadelphia

First published in 2006
by Jessica Kingsley Publishers
116 Pentonville Road
London N1 9JB, UK
and
400 Market Street, Suite 400
Philadelphia, PA 19106, USA

www.jkp.com

Copyright © Jessica Kingsley Publishers 2006
Foreword copyright © Blake Morrison 2006
Printed digitally since 2009

Library of Congress Cataloging in Publication Data
Writing works : a resource handbook for therapeutic writing workshops and activities / edited by Gillie Bolton, Victoria Field, and Kate Thompson ; foreword by Blake Morrison.
    p. cm.
Includes bibliographical references and index.
ISBN-13: 978-1-84310-468-1 (pbk. : alk. paper)
ISBN-10: 1-84310-468-7 (pbk. : alk. paper) 1. Creative writing--Therapeutic use. 2. Psychotherapy. I. Bolton, Gillie. II. Field, Victoria, 1963- III. Thompson, Kate, 1961-
[DNLM: 1. Writing. 2. Psychotherapy--methods. WM 450.5.W9 W957 2006]
RC489.C75W75 2006
616.89'165--dc22

                              2006011613

British Library Cataloguing in Publication Data
A CIP catalogue record for this book is available from the British Library

ISBN 978 1 84310 468 1

Contents

Foreword

'One sheds one's sicknesses in books', D.H. Lawrence wrote after completing *Sons and Lovers*, 'repeats and presents again one's emotions, to be master of them'. Ted Hughes said something similar shortly before he published *Birthday Letters*, a book of elegies to his late wife, Sylvia Plath: 'What's writing really about? It's trying to take fuller possession of the reality of your life – to attack it and attack it and get it under control'. This idea of writing as a way of controlling or mastering one's emotions has sometimes been frowned upon; surely writing ought to be more than therapy, people say. Well, yes, but the process of articulating painful truths can be restorative, healing, even life-saving. And there's no reason why writing produced at moments of crisis or distress can't be good writing, especially if the writer has some guidelines to work with – or a midwife at hand to assist with the birth.

This handbook is written in that spirit, not just to give vague encouragement to would-be writers but as a practical how-to book, with warm-up exercises, tips on how to form and convene writing groups, descriptions of the responsibilities and difficulties involved and countless examples from the pioneering work which the three authors and others have done in this field. There are also personal testimonies from those who have benefited from attending workshops, including, for example, Jane Tozer, who recounts how writing poetry in a little-known verse-form, the ghazal, restored her confidence and 'connected me with intensely personal subject matter'.

The term 'bibliotherapy' has entered the language only recently. But the link between literature and healing goes back to Aristotle and his notion of catharsis (or 'purgation'). Shakespeare, too, understood the importance of self-expression: 'Give sorrow words', he wrote, 'the grief that does not speak/Whispers the o'er fraught heart, and bids it break'.

Giving sorrow words needn't mean pouring things out in a torrent; even confessions have to be shaped. Some poets prefer free verse, but many are liberated by working within a given form or regular rhythmic pattern. Some prose writers are candidly autobiographical, while others boldly invent. There are no hard and fast rules and this book doesn't attempt to legislate. But the exercises it describes – with alphabet poems, acrostics, stories, sonnets, pantoums, fairytales and visualisations – are immensely useful, and whatever your interest in writing, whether you're a counsellor, a teacher or a student, you will find yourself wanting to try them out.

This is a book that deserves a place not just in schools and colleges but in hospitals, prisons, rehab clinics and community centres. Anyone who cares about writing will find it rewarding. And anyone professionally concerned with the health – and mental health – of this country should be made to read it. 'One sheds one's sicknesses in books', as Lawrence said, and this book is part of the cure.

Blake Morrison,
poet, novelist and critic

Around this corner

The afflicted messenger
turning this way and that out of the wind,
passes a window, sees the prisoner,
taps and smiles.

One of them says, I haven't danced enough.

Chairs are lined up along the horizon:
quick, it's that old game, the last to reach them
goes headlong
off the edge of the world.

The prisoner, not looking up,
flicks a fly, spills the mug of tea over the book.

One of them says, an extra-strong hoopla
will keep the dark clouds out.

It's the swimming game now:
be a cupboard flapping open and closed
towards the island
where someone waits.

One of them says, I own a dream
stored in a can.

It's the game of walking into the wall now
as if it's a pillow
and through the pillow
the elusive garden.

One of them says, give me lustre, let slip
a little lustre.

I write this account now we have met again
years later
outside the bakery. Simultaneously
I have handed over half my sandwich
and have received in return half a cake.
Now I am I continuing on, round the bend.

David Hart

Acknowledgements

We would like to thank all the writers who have contributed so generously to *Writing Works*, and the members of Lapidus (The Association for Literary Arts in Personal Development, UK) and the United States' National Association of Poetry Therapy who have contributed so much to the development of work in this field. We are grateful to Jessica Kingsley and Stephen Jones for having faith and belief in our vision for this book, and to Jessica Stevens for her care and support.

Gillie, Victoria and Kate

Gillie Bolton

I would like to express gratitude to all the many professionals, patients, clients and peers with whom I've worked over the last nearly 30 years and from whom I've learned so much: you have taught me nearly all I know in this field. And heartfelt thanks to all my colleagues who've waited patiently (sometimes impatiently) while *Writing Works* has taken priority with my time. Thank you Bill Noble, Richard Meakin, Kate Billingham, Amanda Howe and Sir Kenneth Calman for your faith in my work; Dan Rowland for endlessly sorting out endless computer problems; Alice Rowland for making me perfect boxes for putting things in; and Stephen Rowland for feeding me and making me happy. Finally I would like to thank Victoria and Kate for being stimulating, reliable and enjoyable co-editors.

Victoria Field

I owe a special debt of thanks to the various and vibrant writing communities of Cornwall and the support and friendship of individuals within them – I have learned so much from you all. I would like especially to thank Geri Giebel Chavis and the serendipity of our initial meeting which led to my training as a poetry therapist under her wise and kind supervision. I would also like to thank D.M. Thomas who, in another life, on a distant shore, first introduced me to the idea of a writing workshop and its potential for transformation. Thanks, too, to Gillie and Kate for this opportunity.

Kate Thompson

I owe a debt of gratitude to the many clients and group members I've worked with who have demonstrated what I have believed – that Writing Works; especially S whose dedication was an example to me. I would like to thank Kay Adams who showed me that journal therapy is a professional practice which can be talked about, and under whose auspices I learnt so much. I thank Michael Thompson for keeping me going with encouragement and practical help and for taking the success of this project for read. Thanks also to Robin Thompson for not taking it or me too seriously and for letting me on the computer. And thank you Gillie and Victoria for this rich collaboration.

Introduction

Gillie Bolton, Victoria Field and Kate Thompson

What this Book Offers and Why   *Gillie Bolton*

Supporting and enabling people to find their own way into writing is an art. Writing offers a powerful avenue towards finding out what one thinks, feels, knows, understands, remembers. It can enable fruitful and open exploration of potential thoughts and ideas. If writing can be this illuminating and opening, it can therefore be potentially personally dangerous. Helping people make contact with such essential, deeply vital personal material is, then, a very responsible practice.

Yet, unlike medicine, anyone can do it. There are myriads of writers' groups and individual facilitators of all sorts doing excellent work of encouragement and enablement. Groups are run by writers and writer facilitators, psychological therapists, health professionals such as occupational therapists or nurses, social workers and teachers or tutors. The client group might be called patients, students, service users, participants, clients. And the work happens in community centres, hospitals, schools, colleges, hospices, prisons, substance abuse rehabilitation centres, family medicine centres, and homes. It is undertaken with people from all cultures, with those for whom English is a subsequent language, with the disabled and able-bodied, with the very sick, and with those with few literacy skills.

Writing Works offers a helping hand, guidance and dozens of tried and tested ideas from experienced practitioners for working with writers or would-be writers whatever the setting, and whether in groups or individually. Each exercise gives far more than a writing idea. Each exercise shares the author's experience, knowledge and skill in working with people; each has vital how-to embedded within it.

The activities, exercises or workshops in this collection seem many and varied. They are all very stimulating and can give rise to wonderful, fascinating or personally valuable writing. But they are merely tools to help people to gain contact with their own essential material. Whatever clever, fun or exciting stimulus is used, it is merely a way of enabling people to start writing what they have to write.

The activities in this book are a way of helping to guide people's hands to a doorknob they have not located yet, in a door they have not yet managed to perceive. Once they have their hand on the knob, it's up to them how far they open their own door, how much they allow themselves to experience there and what use they make of it. People write (or do not write) what they want and need to write, whatever we do. We, as facilitators, tutors, therapists, can certainly help. Socrates' dialogic methods have been called *maiutic*: pertaining to midwifery. Since writing has often been likened to giving birth, the metaphor of midwife for the helper-on-the-way is pertinent.

Personal development or therapeutic writing

Group participants, clients or tutees use writing to explore themselves and their situations, to express what they think and feel, and to offer a written record of memories to family and friends. They write for themselves and perhaps a very few significant others, generally retaining authority and complete control. Literary writing, on the other hand, is oriented towards a literary product of as high a quality as possible (in, for example, poetry, fiction, drama) generally aimed at professionally edited publication for an unknown readership.

Therapeutic writing can be the initial stage of literary writing; the ensuing stages of literary crafting, redrafting and editing being focused towards publication. Expressions of private experience are crafted into a public text. The reader of published literature is not primarily interested in the writer but in what the writer has to say. A reader of therapeutic writing, on the whole, responds to the writer as a person, their confidential private expression and their personal development.

What form does it take?

This personal, therapeutic writing could all be called 'journal' or 'diary' writing. These terms mean different things in different contexts; in this book we will use them interchangeably. 'Journal' or 'diary' can be used as an umbrella term to include many different forms of personal writing, such as personal poetry; metaphor exploration and expression; genre story;

personal experience story; unsent letters; dream exploration; dialogues with parts of the body, such as a cancer tumour or an aching tooth; and dialogues with significant fictional, metaphorical figures such as my internal critic (see below), or my child self.

Personal journal, diary or first draft writing can have an intensely cathartic or gently illuminative effect upon the writer. Some such writings can also form effective communication aids between writer and relatives, friends or clinicians: there are certain things which cannot be said, but they can be written.

Literary forms such as novels, sonnets or plays might form part of the personal writing repertoire, or they might not. This is because personal writing is not aimed at publication beyond a small group or family and friends. Sometimes it is not read by anyone else, occasionally not even the writer (who may even gain cathartic relief by burning or ripping the text). It is not the form that matters, but rather the process and act of writing and the content, and the impact of that content on the writer and perhaps some personally related readers. Form can offer specific benefit, however, to some writers (see Chapter 5).

How to enable and support personal writers is fully covered and exemplified in this book's varied activities and exercises.

Writing for publication

Writing for publication can be therapeutic or personally developing. This can take writers and their tutors by surprise. Many people join a class to write to publish, because they assume this is what writing is about. Yet once they start writing they are taken by the powerful tide of the process to learn more about themselves and their situation. An awareness of this is vital for any creative writing tutor in any setting, whether it be a university or a holiday course. These tutors or lecturers need to understand that at times they will need to care for the *writer* as a person, rather than solely for the development of the *writing*. Sometimes they may need to seek supervision or advice.

The processes of *redrafting* can also be intensely personally informative. Redrafting can be a process of trying to get as close as possible to the images or narratives in the mind. Many deeply painful or problematic memories can only be accessed through metaphor. Writing, due to the way it powerfully wields metaphor, can allow access to these otherwise hidden memories. Redrafting can be a process of gently perceiving and understanding these metaphorically based memories more and more clearly.

The internal critic

The success of our joint ventures into these unknown worlds is deeply affected by the critic inside every one of our clients or group participants (and us). We are all made up of a host of different elements; it's these different voices we listen to in writing. I have often called these the different hats we wear at different times of our daily lives; the stern critic is one of them. At its best this critic is deeply constructive, enabling writers to gain a critical distance in order to redraft effectively, to see where writing doesn't quite work and how to develop it so it comes closer to doing what we want it to do.

Only too often, however, this critic is deeply destructive. One name for it is writer's block. Ted Hughes metaphorically called it a policeman, poet Dorothy Nimmo a black parrot on her shoulder; Virginia Woolf saw it as the angel in the house who tried to persuade her to be a real woman only concerned with domestic matters. Many people locate their critic as a head teacher putting a red pen through everything creative. This critic is the one who whispers in your ear that you are a rubbish writer: who are you to write? Sometimes it even prevents your pen from meeting the paper, your fingers from even touching the keys.

Facilitators, tutors or therapists can help deal with this destructive influence, sometimes even turning it to good. There are specific exercises in this book to enable people to put a spotlight on their critic, dialogue with it perhaps in order to listen and respond constructively to it. Something that is understood (even if only partially) and that you begin to tackle is part-way to being dealt with. I say part-way – these internal critics are immensely powerful beasts with myriads of different snapping heads: chop off one and ten more might sprout, all breathing fire. Last week I used a metaphor exercise like the Furniture Game to help a group of doctor writers name their critic. That is, if the critic were a, say, animal, country, piece of furniture and so on, what would he or she be? I then asked them to write a letter to whichever metaphor seemed most apt (one had a tiger), and their own reply. They scribbled furiously for half an hour, finding the exercise powerfully useful.

Foundations

There are a range of essential foundations to this work. Facilitator and group or client all being as clear as possible about their joint aims and objectives is essential. Some time needs to be spent initially gently sorting these out, and ensuring people have a similar enough attitude to what they're doing, and what they hope to get out of the exercise. In a one-to-one situation this could be called a contract between therapist/ facilitator and client. Boundaries and ground rules need to be established.

Confidentiality, trust, respect, pacing, boundaries; how to introduce writing effectively and safely enough; who owns what, and so on, are all vital areas to be considered initially. Only once these foundations are in place should a facilitator embark on any of the activities described.

A vital, yet insignificant, word in thinking about essential foundations to this work is 'enough'. The set-up should feel safe enough to participants and facilitator. If it's too safe, and everyone writes about safe issues, nothing will happen and they'll all soon stop in discouragement. Facilitators should feel confident enough of what they're doing, and the writers need to be self-aware enough, brave and daring enough and yet secure enough in the space the facilitator is holding for them. People like dangerous sports to a greater or a lesser degree, but most people don't undertake them knowing they're suicidal – such sports are safe and dangerous enough.

Trust and respect are also key. Writer and facilitator trusting and respecting each other is a requisite, as is writer and facilitator trusting and respecting the processes in which they are engaged. Writing is an eminently trustworthy process if it is undertaken with respect.

Not only is the process of writing to be handled with respect, so also is every writer's writing. Every writer is the authority of their own writing. In this kind of work, the writer will always write the right thing. It is impossible to get it wrong. Writers are the authority of themselves and their own experience, knowledge, thoughts, feelings, memories and dreams. This vital issue makes this work different from teaching. I am no more authoritative than any of the writers with whom I work, whether medical consultant or asylum-seeker teenager. What they write is incontrovertibly theirs, and they have complete authority over and about it. As personal development facilitator or supervisor or tutor I can support and advise on processes used, and help people face and stay with whatever they need to. I have no authority concerning editing or redrafting their writing, unless they specifically invite me to step out of my personal development relationship, and invite me to put on my teacher or editor's hat.

'Fun' and 'enjoyment' are other keywords. Nothing of excitement, interest or usefulness will happen if writer and facilitator are not enjoying themselves, because writing is an utterly enjoyable activity in its own right. More than that even: it can be obsessively hypnotic. Once started it can be hard to stop. Any writer will say that the really odd and exciting thing about writing is that it develops a life of its own. You have to continue writing to see what the characters are going to say, where the poetic images will take you, and to find out what happens. And you never do find out what happens in the end because, rather like climbing a mountain, what appears as the end (or the top) turns out to be just a landmark on the way. There are always further tantalisingly not-quite-in-focus areas to explore just ahead. The more you write the more you want to write, and the more you discover and learn.

The satisfaction and thrill of creating something which wasn't there before is like no other. What must it have felt like to sense Elizabeth Bennett, Hamlet or Bilbo Baggins becoming living breathing beings under their creators' pens? The very creative process is deeply self-affirming and creating of self-confidence: I've made this; therefore I really exist and am worth something!

The difference between this and mountain- or rock-climbing is that there are no maps or guides showing specific ways to go, pointing out the dangers and the glories. Every word is a new exploration for every writer. *Writing Works* offers them guidance and support at least.

Running Groups   *Victoria Field*

This section is intended to be a guide to tackling some of the practical issues of running a therapeutic writing group. Of course, practicalities cannot easily be separated from the content of the sessions – being part of a writing group is very much an holistic experience.

Writing has been compared to fire – it can release energy, lead to catharsis and healing; it can be warming and comforting but it is also possible to be burned or even destroyed by it. The writing process should be treated with the same respect with which we treat fire – it is a valuable resource if properly harnessed. In particular, anyone setting out to run a group, first and foremost, must ensure the safety – in every sense – of those who join.

That said, what follows is not intended to be rigidly prescriptive – groups have their own magic and chemistry, and a skilled facilitator, whilst well prepared, will always be ready to work with what comes up, which may well be surprising. Most facilitators have had the experience of using an exercise or activity with one group successfully only for it to be poorly received on another occasion. What exactly 'happens' in a therapeutic writing group is complex and much of it is unconscious or barely conscious. In most of the accounts of workshops in this book, facilitators have chosen to give only the observable details – that is, 'I did this, they did that'. Others have added commentary about how it felt for participants, based on self-reports. Beneath these two kinds of experience is a whole dynamic of motivations, transferences, projections and changing social norms that inform both the writing and the therapeutic process.

Therapeutic writing does not necessarily happen in groups: many people discover for themselves the benefits of keeping a diary, 'splurging' onto the page or engaging in what are sometimes called 'morning pages' (recommended by Julia Cameron, 1994, and Dorothea Brande, 1996) to clear the mind at the beginning of the day. Such writing need never be read by another person, not even by the writer. Writing for oneself in this way can be extremely valuable but may lead to an entrenchment of ideas, attitudes or feelings. Outside listeners or readers can offer insight or challenges that may lead to the writer seeing new possibilities for change or development. For example, there may be someone who has a tendency to write poems in the second person, addressing either a specific or generalised 'you' – sometimes, this may indicate a distancing of emotions and a suggestion that they try writing in the first person might yield interesting insights.

There are also therapists and counsellors who may encourage their clients to engage in writing of various kinds to be shared on a one-to-one basis. Here, the writing forms part of a more general therapeutic intervention and is not usually the primary therapy on offer.

For the purposes of this section, it is assumed that a group is coming together specifically to engage in writing as a primary activity or therapy.

Context

There is often a resistance to the use of the word 'therapy' in conjunction with an arts activity. It can be argued that all writing is therapeutic in that, like walking, gardening, painting or cooking, it can enable us to transcend our immediate state for a while whilst engaging in a satisfying activity. However, there is growing evidence that writing provides some unique benefits for mental and physical health. The pioneer in this field is James Pennebaker (1997) whose book *Opening Up* provided some of the first empirical evidence of these benefits.

It is perhaps helpful to see a continuum from 'writing for pleasure or recreation' (which may be 'therapeutic') to writing which is explicitly undertaken as 'therapy'. The context of the writing group and the expectations – both explicit and not – of the participants will probably indicate where on the continuum a particular group comes.

A straightforward creative writing group, in, for example, adult education or a public library, may well lead to participants sharing or drawing on personal experience. Here I would suggest that, whilst exploring personal material may be therapeutic, the genesis of a piece of writing is to some extent incidental and a tutor or facilitator would usually keep their focus on the writing as writing rather than personal expression. It is hoped that the tutor will be alert enough to acknowledge the use of personal material – especially when it might be sensitive – but in the context of what the student wants to achieve with their own writing. A parallel example is provided by one particular Poetry Group in the south of England that takes the form of an open workshop focusing on rigorous criticism – here, even though poems may be brought that are clearly based on personal experience, the discussion is likely to revolve around line breaks, punctuation and metre. There are clearly drawn boundaries between the writing as an artistic object and the writer. In both cases, it is expected that the writer has some emotional distance from their writing.

The kind of language used to describe a particular group reflects its ethos. The terms 'tutor' (instructor) and 'student' imply learning about a topic and that there is a body of knowledge to be conveyed. Such a group can be indirectly therapeutic. For example, Dominic McLoughlin, an experienced counsellor and poet, runs poetry groups in hospices where he clearly identifies himself as a 'tutor' and the students are there to learn more about poetry for its own sake – as a literary object rather than a tool for exploring their situation. David Hart, a poet with wide experience in psychiatric and health settings, always calls himself a poet and insists that it is the quality of writing produced that is paramount in his sessions.

Some writing groups may be more explicitly therapeutic. This might be conveyed by a course title, for example 'Writing for Well-Being' or

'Writing for Self-Discovery'; or else by virtue of their location or client group – for example, a writing group for people in recovery or in day treatment for mental health problems. Here, the emphasis is on writing as process and writing as a tool for exploring personal issues. The group convenor or leader is likely to be called a 'facilitator' or 'practitioner' rather than a 'tutor', and group members might be termed 'participants' or 'patients'. The terminology again is important. In such groups, the literary merit or otherwise of the writing produced is less important than the content of writing and its significance to its writer. There is often an emphasis on spontaneous writing even though pieces may later be revised and redrafted.

In some cases, what is on offer is explicitly bibliotherapy, writing therapy or poetry therapy. Here, attending a writing group might be part of a person's treatment programme and they are likely to have been referred to the group by a GP, psychiatrist or occupational therapist. The emphasis is on using writing to further more general treatment goals, perhaps related to social interaction, self-awareness and self-esteem, and the therapist will work as part of a team, usually in a 'medicalised' context. For members of such a group, this clear focus can be an advantage or disadvantage. I worked for a year with a woman who had a diagnosis of severe and enduring mental illness. She discharged herself from the poetry therapy group I ran in a day treatment centre, and then enrolled on my adult education 'Writing for Self-Discovery' course where her diagnosis was never disclosed nor an issue. Conversely, the closed nature of a therapy group means that participants who are sometimes extremely unwell can still attend and, whilst they may not be able to speak at all, derive benefit from others' discussion and the structure offered by a group they have come to know and trust.

There are areas of middle ground. There are, for example, library-based writing groups which are open to all but the publicity states that people with 'mental health problems are especially welcome'. This sends the message that, whilst no one has to disclose any psychiatric history, the facilitator and other group members will not be fazed by any reference to it.

Contract and ground rules
A contract between the facilitator and participants can be formal or informal. It is basically a mutual understanding of what each side expects from the other.

In an educational setting, this is sometimes imposed and students may have to state their 'learning objectives'. In other groups, especially where there is open enrolment, the facilitator will usually invite participants to say why they are there and their hopes and expectations for the group. It is interesting to note these and reflect them back at the end of the session or course – participants often find that they have achieved quite different objectives.

It is always appropriate for the facilitator to introduce themselves, the purpose of the session or course and what the ethos is. If the group is meeting outside a clinical setting, it is also essential to draw clear boundaries. For example, I would say to an adult education or writers' group that, whilst I would want them to write authentically about issues of importance, this is not 'therapy' and that participants are expected to manage their own material; that if a topic is 'too hot to handle' then it should be saved for another more appropriate place, perhaps one-to-one psychotherapy. However, I also make it clear that it is perfectly permissible to cry during a session (this is often an unexpressed fear of many people beginning to write). In my experience, tears are most likely in response to another group member's writing and are testimony to human empathy.

A personal choice in a therapeutic writing setting is my decision to make it clear to participants that I will not be commenting on the literary quality or potential for publication of any work produced. I also don't read it on the page – all work shared is read aloud. Keeping sharing oral also means that literacy skills such as spelling and punctuation are not an issue. It helps to emphasise writing as 'process' where whatever is written is valid and not yet 'fixed'. There is nothing, of course, to prevent the writing being developed or used elsewhere.

In a therapeutic writing group in a clinical setting, the purpose of the writing is explicitly to facilitate self-awareness. This may be by examining issues that are extremely serious, such as suicide, sexual or other abuse, chronic depression or psychotic symptoms. The difference here is that the therapist has the back-up of supervision and access to the key worker responsible for a particular patient. They will usually, too, have had extensive information about individuals in the group and a chance to talk to them beforehand. Sometimes, group members find it easier to write than speak and, in one clinical group I worked with, whilst spontaneous writing was encouraged and shared during the sessions, some members would write poems in the interim week addressing what had been discussed in the previous session. These individuals were very withdrawn and one of the objectives for me was to encourage them to express themselves directly as well as in writing – however, without the poems, I would never have known what feelings and questions were emerging from the sessions.

The question of ground rules needs to be considered, even if they are not all explicitly stated. Sometimes, the facilitator will be clear what these should be and on other occasions it might be appropriate to develop them in conjunction with the group members. Sometimes, basic courtesy and consideration for other members can be assumed; when working with other groups, especially perhaps those including young people or people in recovery, the need for these might have to be made explicit. Problem issues might include absence, persistent lateness, cigarette breaks or a group member who dominates the discussion – all of which can be useful to discuss.

One ground rule that must be explicitly stated, and periodically restated, is that of confidentiality – that the personal affairs of group members should not be discussed outside. This is essential in establishing an environment where people feel free to disclose and to write freely.

In terms of responding to the writing of participants, I have found it useful to suggest that the most valuable response is attentive listening and reflecting back on what kind of feeling the writing engendered in the listener. Members of the group should refrain from making qualitative judgements unless invited to do so by the writer.

Facilitator qualities and qualifications

This is a complicated area – facilitators come from a whole variety of professional backgrounds or none. Part of the excitement of this new area of work is that there is currently no one route into it, but this also makes it difficult for employers and potential host institutions to know that a facilitator has the appropriate training and qualities to lead a therapeutic writing group.

Lapidus (the Association for Literary Arts in Personal Development) has produced a document outlining the 'core competencies' that can reasonably be expected of facilitators. This is available to members from its website (www.lapidus.org.uk). The competencies outlined include a commitment to both their own writing and the therapeutic process. They should have some experience of managing a group and working in a team and some training in counselling techniques, as well as a knowledge of appropriate literary materials. There should also be clear evidence that they are committed to their ongoing personal and professional development. NAPT (the National Association for Poetry Therapy) requires a background in psychology and literature for admission to its training programmes.

More difficult to assess are the personal qualities that enable a facilitator to work in an intuitive way that respects group members and actively fosters personal development and growth. An essential part of this is self-knowledge and a clear sense of boundaries. Facilitators need to be very aware of their own areas of vulnerability and to ensure that they build regular supervision into their practice.

For those who may be new to this work but feel that they have something to offer, my advice would be to attend as many workshops as possible and then to begin perhaps by shadowing or assisting someone with experience or volunteering under the supervision of someone with appropriate training.

If seeking paid employment, insurance and Criminal Records Board clearance are usually required. Advice on this and recommended rates of pay may be obtained from arts education and arts and health agencies.

Practicalities

Environmental factors are very important for any group but perhaps especially for a therapeutic writing group. A clean, quiet, comfortable, well-ventilated room with easy access to refreshments and toilets and adequate space for the number of people is essential. So too is the basic structure of a session – starting and finishing on time, breaks at regular intervals, not having too many or too few people in the group and giving everyone an equal opportunity to speak all contribute to the well-being of the group. Consistency is especially important in a clinical setting where anxiety over external factors can prevent full participation.

Some groups feel most comfortable sitting at tables, others on easy chairs. In warm weather, it is sometimes possible to have some sessions outside but this often leads to a lack of focus, difficulty hearing or concentrating and physical discomfort for some people. A compromise could be having the group discussion indoors and for the writing part of the session to be done wherever individuals feel most at ease.

Content of the session

This entire book makes suggestions for the possible content of a therapeutic writing session. Planning should be done bearing in mind such factors as the client group and the nature of the session. Questions to ask include: is it a one-off or an open-ended group, or is it part of a course? Do the group members know each other well or is it a new group? *Biblio/Poetry Therapy*, the classic textbook by Hynes and Hynes Berry (1994), provides useful analysis for planning sessions.

Most sessions will include introductions, a recap, if appropriate, some kind of warm-up activity and then some more extended writing followed by sharing of the writing and discussion. The writing might be stimulated by a text introduced by the facilitator or maybe through so-called *realia* brought in, for example objects from nature, buttons, postcards. Again, the terminology used by the facilitator should be appropriate to the group. The word 'exercise' is commonly used in writing workshops and has connotations of practising an art or physiotherapy. It also, for many people, invokes school and possibly unhappy experiences in formal education. 'Activity' is less loaded but is perhaps patronising, implying young children. It is possible to avoid both words by inviting or suggesting that participants might want to 'do some writing' or 'make a poem'.

When it comes to reading back or sharing work, whilst facilitators should encourage full participation, it is important to allow people to pass if they wish. Sometimes, the suggestion that they read just a little or one sentence might enable someone reticent to contribute. It is often in the reading back that the most intense part of the session occurs – being truly listened to is a rare experience for many of us and to be listened to attentively and respectfully can be very empowering.

It is usually recommended that the facilitator joins in the writing with the participants, so demonstrating the value of the activity. There are differing opinions about whether the facilitator should read back their writing. My own feeling, from a perspective both as a group member and a facilitator, is that the task of the facilitator is to be attentive and to hold the group and it is impossible to do this and engage in therapeutic writing at the same time. Reading back also takes time which could be spent on the group members. If I am facilitating, I always write; but I do so fairly superficially and do not volunteer to read back except on the rare occasions that a group member asks me to.

Time management is vital to ensure that there is space for people to say what they need to say and for the session to close appropriately. This is especially important when people may have been writing from a very deep place and possibly accessed some difficult thoughts and feelings. The facilitator should ensure that everyone is ready to go out into the world again from the safe confines of the group.

Problem solving

In the life of any group there will be challenges. Sometimes, especially when buried feelings are being accessed for the first time, participants may complain about the group or the facilitator – projecting feelings of discomfort onto them. The facilitator should be detached enough not to take criticism personally but to address it in the context of the group.

Another common occurrence is a member attempting to dominate the group even to the extent of undermining the facilitator. This can often be tackled by reference to ground rules allowing everyone the option of equal time and by acknowledging that the facilitator does not have privileged knowledge.

There will be times when it may no longer be appropriate for someone to continue to attend a therapeutic writing group. This may be due to disruptive behaviour or because symptoms have become worrying, especially if someone has psychotic episodes. Here, supervision is essential so that steps can be taken to ensure the continuing well-being of both the individual and the group as a whole. Irvin Yalom's (1985) classic book on group psychotherapy, *The Theory and Practice of Group Psychotherapy*, has much that is directly applicable to writing groups and is highly recommended for an insight into group dynamics.

Self-care

Finally, in order to give effectively to others, it is vital that the facilitator takes time to rest and regenerate.

Writing Therapeutically and Writing in Therapy

Kate Thompson

That writing can be therapeutic is something we take as axiomatic in this volume and is amply demonstrated in the variety of contributions we present. It is something we know from our own experience, from observation and from the responses of those in our groups or clients in one-to-one sessions. It is perhaps useful, for both facilitators and participants, to make a distinction between:

1. a therapeutic writing group

2. a writing group with therapeutic outcomes

3. writing in therapy.

However, it is not always possible to make discrete categories, for, even in creative writing groups with no expected or intended therapeutic benefit or outcome, such as many in adult education settings, the process of writing can let loose strange insights and emotions. The unwary facilitator can be taken by surprise and may possibly not have given much thought to boundaries and appropriate responses to the situation in which someone, perhaps for the first time, gives voice to deep emotion or memories.

Writing and the relationship with the self

By inviting clients to explore the idea of writing, we are offering them a way of working which goes beyond the confines of the therapeutic relationship and returns them to the relationship with the self in a direct and immediate way. For example, in journal therapy the primary focus is on developing intimacy with the self. This can be a powerful way of dealing with feelings of shame which can be at the root of much resistance to doing therapeutic work. Writing can be a way of uncovering the unacknowledged or recovering the repressed. For some people writing will be the first stage in therapeutic work and will allow them then to speak about things which are too painful or too shameful to be addressed directly even in the safe space of the therapeutic relationship.

The privacy of writing, whether it is in a handwritten journal, on a computer or on scraps of paper, can be the first step in sharing something with another person, for example a therapist or significant other. Writing within therapy can be done before, during or after sessions with a therapist. Clients may choose to share their writing with their therapist in different ways and for different reasons – someone may read it to the therapist or, perhaps when it is too painful to say, ask the therapist to read it either silently or aloud; or writing may be sent to the therapist before a session.

A client who was uncovering her history of sexual abuse in therapy with me needed me to know things but was utterly unable to speak about them. She was literally unvoiced, so would e-mail me her writing before each session so that I 'knew' and had witnessed the story. Eventually she became able to read to me what she had written and finally to be able to speak in a direct and unmediated way. Writing was her way of recovering her voice.

When writing is part of the therapeutic contract, issues such as how much time will be spent on reading clients' writing outside of sessions or what sort of response to e-mails is expected are all part of the contract which needs to be negotiated.

Writing within therapy

The relationship between therapist and client is crucial in writing within therapy. Increasingly research tells us this relationship is the most significant factor in the progress and outcome of therapy, rather than the type of therapy or the orientation of the therapist. Whilst writing therapy is not yet a stand-alone therapy like art therapy, music therapy or drama therapy, some psychological therapists introduce writing into their work with clients and interest in writing as a tool of therapy is growing (Wright 2005). Therapeutic modalities such as cognitive behavioural therapy or cognitive analytic therapy use particular forms of writing as part of the therapeutic plan.

Safety and ethical considerations

The safety of the client is paramount in the therapeutic relationship. Therapists are bound by ethical frameworks to ensure safe practice. Writing is a powerful tool which in some circumstances can threaten the ego boundaries of some clients.

There is one activity which can produce astonishing and creative results but can also have disturbing outcomes and should be used with caution. This is the technique known as freewriting or writing in flow. When the mind is let loose to roam the undergrowth of the unconscious it can produce unexpected results and it can let loose demons. Pacing and structure in writing therapy are vital to give clients the containment they need. The eventual aim is for clients to become self-pacing in their therapeutic writing.

All practitioners have a duty of care to their students or clients. Many settings will provide practitioners with regulations, frameworks or requirements by which they are bound, and these are intended to keep practitioners and clients safe. In this book we have a wide range of examples of different kinds of structured exercises; in some the structure is so light that it is hardly apparent and yet it provides containment for those who need it. We see very vulnerable groups of people responding to the exercises in ways that allow them to begin to experience healing and growth, and to begin to take control of their own process.

Therapeutic writing research

The therapeutic benefit of expressive writing is an area which is beginning to accrue significant research interest and evidence. In the US James Pennebaker (1997) has been conducting trials for several years to look at the effects of writing on emotional and physical well-being and the health benefits of expressive writing. In *The Writing Cure* (Lepore and Smyth 2002) a range of international authors describe their attempts to discover how and why writing affects health. In the UK there is growing interest from writers, therapists and scientist-practitioners in the use of writing as a therapeutic medium (Bolton *et al.* 2002). From whichever angle people approach there are some common factors to be considered.

Writing groups with therapeutic outcomes

Writing groups with therapeutic outcomes are those which have an explicitly personal development aim and act as support group for the participants. In these it is generally accepted that there will be some level of personal revelation and disclosure and so issues of confidentiality need to be made explicit and discussed in the ground rules at the beginning of the group.

It is perhaps also useful to think about contact outside the group and whether this should be discussed and brought back into the group. If contact is not disclosed it can cause envy and rivalrous dynamics within the group.

Some groups of this kind have been going for years and participants develop a great degree of intimacy and involvement which can be tremendously enriching both for them and for the facilitator. The dynamics of the group, the relationships which develop within the group and between the group and the facilitator, are powerful aspects of and contributors to the therapeutic benefit of the writing.

Dealing with distressed group members
Boundaries are something to be negotiated in groups at the outset and this may include what to do when someone becomes upset. It is almost inevitable that this will occur at some time in the life of a group. People can be taken by surprise by something in another group member's writing which evokes memories or feelings or startles them into making connections between things in their own lives or seeing things in a different way. On other occasions group members can be reminded of relationships from their own lives by other people in the group which can have emotional results.

It is useful to think about what to do when a group member becomes upset or overwhelmed in a meeting or perhaps rushes *distraught* from the room; probably this will occur at some time and not necessarily in the most obvious group or with the participant one might have expected. If someone does leave the room it is probably because they want to put some distance between what is happening for them in the room and the other people and this should be respected. It is of course important to ensure they are safe but also to manage the safety of the group as a whole which will have been disturbed by such a dramatic event. Course facilitators can be unsure of what to do and may even think it is not their responsibility to deal with emotion and chaos.

In such circumstances it is often a good idea to wait before doing anything, to offer reassurance first to the group, which will look to the facilitator for guidance (the facilitator may have assumed the role of the reassuring parent for the group). Only when the facilitator is sure that the group is functioning, perhaps writing again, should they leave the room and attend to the absenter, perhaps gently saying something like: 'Take the time you need, come back when you are ready.'

If the participant needs to go home then it is important to make it possible for them to return the following week without embarrassment. In some groups members may form friendships and alliances, in which case there may be someone from within the group who is a more appropriate person to attend to the absentee; this leaves the facilitator to concentrate on holding the group.

Supervision and the facilitator's emotional process
Psychological therapists are required to have regular supervision as part of their practice in order to maintain their professional accreditation.

Supervision, either in a group or in a one-to-one relationship, gives them access to a space in which they can discuss distressing and difficult material which may arise in the work with clients and to explore their own thoughts and feelings. This allows them to reflect on any issues which may be evoked for them by their clients and to investigate how this affects the work.

In writing groups the group facilitator is not immune from 'affect' in the group; just as a participant may be disturbed by something which comes up in someone's writing, so might the facilitator. The facilitator has the added responsibility of holding the group dynamics and may find it beneficial to try and think about this with a supervisor. Supervision is a place where boundaries can be investigated and process, content and relationships can be synthesised.

Supervision becomes an essential part of the practice, providing a relationship in which the practitioner can be supported and helped to understand the process of the work. It should be provided to or sought by those who are working with writing where clients begin to reveal personal issues of significance.

Writing in supervision

Bringing writing into the supervisory process is another version of writing in therapy. As a supervisor I encourage supervisees to write about their own thoughts and feelings and reflections on therapy as a method of self-supervision, thereby harnessing the power of writing to deepen the therapeutic work. Again, this is about the relationship with the self, or between parts of the self (for example between the professional therapist self and the over-protective mother self), as distinct from writing case notes or supervision presentations; it is deeply personal writing.

Note

All contributors to *Writing Works* have given written permission for the inclusion of their work. Some names and details have been altered for confidentiality.

PART ONE

Writing from Without

CHAPTER I

Warming Up and Working Together

Edited by Kate Thompson

Beginnings are exciting, shot through with the adrenaline of the new and fuelled by expectation. They are also frightening and anxiety provoking and full of uncertainty, states which we go to great lengths to avoid. They are both the agent and product of change and change is, by its very nature, always disturbing. When people attend their first workshop or attempt their first piece of therapeutic writing, on their own or at another's instigation, it is often a result of change or an attempt to accomplish change.

The beginning of a course, a session, a workshop arouses many thoughts and feelings in participants and facilitator alike. Many of the contributors to this book allude to the anxiety provoked by the prospect of sharing private things in personal writing springing from unknown places. In this chapter Victoria Field recalls her own anxiety as a participant in her first writing workshop. This acts as a timely reminder to all of us engaged in this work that our own experiences are a vital tool. Her exercise here suggests no sharing of writing but initial conversational sharing as a way of coming together and overcoming some of those fears. Participants then introduce their partner to the whole group but their writing and themselves are kept private.

Writing may be an unfamiliar idiom, may even be unavailable to some – as in Kate D'Lima's piece, where people are helped by others to tell their stories which the group recognises and collaborates upon. Zeeba Ansari talks about expectations and the failure of expectation: anxiety and expectation are all tied up together at the start of anything new.

So, how to begin? Warm-ups are those exercises designed as preliminaries, intended to warm the ink in the pen, melt the resistance, and reduce the level of anxiety in the room and in the person. They need to be short and clear, containing without being prescriptive (often what people need at this stage is to be reassured that they cannot 'do it wrong').

I have a favourite activity which I often do even before introductions or ground rules. This is so people can establish relationship with the self and with writing before they have to interact or share. I offer the following questions for a three-minute write:

> Who am I?
>
> Why am I here?
>
> What do I want?

These questions produce answers on many levels and evoke different responses depending on time or context. I then invite people to read and give themselves written feedback, before sharing with the group their thoughts and feelings about the process or the writing itself, should they want. (Adapted from an exercise in a workshop with Kathleen Adams.)

There are other ways of beginning apart from engaging instantly with writing. Victoria Field uses a structured conversational game to break the ice and allow people to begin to make connections with other members without exposure. Cheryl Moskowitz describes beginning with other kinds of activity, going out of the room, walking through other spaces and becoming aware of the environment through sensory experience.

In simplicity we often return to childlike states when we would hope to have been safe and protected. Some contributors make this link and Larry Butler's exercise invites people to think about their fears and expectations at the beginning of a workshop using the acrostic form (where the letters of a word, often a name, are written down the page to provide the first letter of each line) which is often familiar from childhood. He calls the acrostic 'a great leveller' suggesting that all participants are equal within the form. Kathleen Adams takes the connection to childhood one step further in her AlphaPoems which she explicitly links to the rhythms of early years and psychodynamic psychotherapy theory.

In beginnings a facilitator can take the opportunity to establish cohesiveness in the room: relationships begin to build internally for individuals and externally trust begins to grow within the group. Research has shown that group cohesiveness is correlated with positive therapeutic outcome (Yalom 1985), just as the relationship is shown to be the most significant factor in individual work. Initially, as Yalom says, 'you [the facilitator] are the group's primary unifying force; the members relate to one another at first through their common relationship to you' (Yalom 1985, p.113).

Cheryl Moskowitz thinks about the wonder of this process and looks at different ways of being and writing together and of facilitating the journey towards cohesiveness.

Kathleen Adams first establishes a safe group experience in her workshop from which people can then move with some confidence into their own individual space and writing. Kate D'Lima moves the other way: from individual to absorption and acceptance by the group.

Where are you Today?   *Victoria Field*

This idea has evolved from the old writing workshop favourite – the Furniture Game (in which people are asked to choose a metaphor for a person such as an animal, flower or piece of furniture). It provides an oral route into therapeutic writing and is a great ice-breaker with a group of strangers at the beginning of a new course. Depending on the size of the group and how much discussion there is at the end, this takes around 45 minutes.

At five minutes to one, I walk into the large, light room at the back of the Arts Centre. The tables are arranged in a horseshoe shape and between 12 and 18 people are seated around them. There is a mixture of apprehension and excitement in the air. It is the first session of a ten-week course in 'Writing for Self-Discovery' and I, as the tutor, am also excited and nervous at the prospect of the journey ahead. Today, we are complete strangers – after ten weeks, several will comment that they know their fellow students better than their own family.

All I have from the adult education college before this first session is a list of names and addresses. I see that most students are local but am always surprised at how some are prepared to travel many miles. There are usually four or five female names to every male. This is an afternoon course and, typically, those attending will have paid a concessionary fee indicating that they are retired, students or claiming benefits. Of the others, some will be shift or part-time workers or else looking after school-age children. One year, the ages ranged from 18 to 88.

I have no idea how much writing the students will have done – only that it will vary hugely. Having attended my own first creative workshop less than ten years ago, I do know how daunting it is to share one's personal writing. I also know that some will have had unhappy experiences in formal education, and attending a 'class', with the possibility of being judged, takes enormous courage. It helps that this course is held in a busy arts centre in the middle of town, rather than on school or college premises. All of these issues will be addressed directly later in this first session when I introduce my aims for the course, its emphasis on 'process' and the fact that I will not be reading their work on the page.

I have two intentions with this activity – to hear everyone's voice, both literal and imaginative, and to have everyone write something unexpected that will confirm to them that they 'can do it'.

I begin by asking people to sit comfortably and focus on their breathing, closing their eyes if they wish. To relax. I then ask them to answer what may seem an odd question – if they were a place, what place would they be? I say, it may be a whole country, a city, a village, a piece of countryside or a building. I encourage them to stay with their first thought and then to consider the place from different perspectives – is it busy or quiet? Old, new or a mixture? What is the climate like? What is it like visually? What is its history? And so on. I check whether everyone has somewhere.

I then ask people to pair up and find a space with someone to whom they have not spoken yet and to introduce themselves as the place. 'I am Patricia – I am Petersburg' or 'I am Michael – I am Swanpool Beach'. Their partner is then to ask them questions as if they are the place. 'How do you feel about being so cold in winter?' or 'What's it like when all the tourists come?'.

I allow ten minutes for this, announcing, after five minutes, that if one of the pair has dominated the partners should swap over to allow equal time for each of them. I am aware that some pairs stay with the metaphor and use the first person, whilst others begin to discuss the places in a general way. Yet others will discover other common ground and begin to chat. I don't think this matters.

I then ask them to return to their seats and to introduce their partner with their place and to say just one or two things that came out of their conversation. 'This is Betty – she is Southern Spain, hot and passionate'. 'This is Sally – she is a tiny Yorkshire village, remote and quiet'. Often, fellow students will express surprise and delight as the places mentioned somehow enter the room and change the atmosphere.

I then invite reflections on doing that activity. These often include how it gives a short cut to understanding the person; how places, like people, are complex and changing and how it was fun to use a metaphor. I suggest that, on different days, we might well choose completely different places.

I then invite everyone just to write a few lines in their notebook – for themselves only – on the place they chose, its characteristics and anything they may have learned about themselves as a result.

Everyone's voice has been heard by everyone in the group and everyone has written something.

This activity can stand alone as an ice-breaker but is also a natural lead-in to other variations of the Furniture Game, where other metaphors (plants, animals, furniture) can be used to describe people.

Hobnobs   *Angie Butler*

Hobnob is a meeting of a small supportive group of people with an interest in writing, often around a kitchen table, sometimes outside. The sessions will differ, but may be led by one or two members of the group, sharing ideas or starting points for writing. There is always coffee and biscuits and often cake and laughter.

Begin by choosing a familiar saying or proverb – it could be the title of a song that can't leave you alone.

'Time and tide waits for no man'

'And cry salt tears'

'Every cloud has a silver lining'

Use each word to start a poem, rather like an acrostic. Repeat each word.

Time...

Time...

And...

And...

Tide...

Tide...

Waits...

Waits...

You could end with the whole phrase or some of the words for the last line. It is good to do as a warm-up as it gives a structure, but the 'rules' can be broken if better ideas or words seem appropriate.

> And cry salt tears
> And the boy from the sea met the girl of the sea
> And they loved, passionately, deeply, swimmingly
> And they thought of their future
>
> Cry for the pain of separation
> Cry for the pain of love
> Cry for the happiness they found in each other
>
> Salt in the wounds of parting
> Salt of the tears they tasted
> Salt from the seas that separate
>
> Tears as they thought of their future
> Tears for the pain of love
> Tears tearing their souls
>
> And they cried, and they cried salt tears.

The Magician's Assistant   *Zeeba Ansari*

Imagine a diverse group of people sitting around a kitchen table. Imagine their peer-group nerves, their expectations and their fear of the unknown. Particularly the creative unknown.

The setting was a local Lapidus group, 'Hobnob' – an informal monthly get-together of practitioners, creative writers and writer-practitioners – at the home of one of the group members. We had agreed that the meeting, lasting two and a half hours, would centre around a poetry workshop – joy for some, horror for others, particularly those who had never written poetry before. I was one of two facilitators who had constructed a series of exercises designed to stimulate experienced writers and beginners alike. The theme of the workshop was Magic Words, and the context was the symbiotic relationship between the arts and personal development. We were there to make words magic, but also to explore the issues thrown up by the creative process into the material it produced.

The exercise I'd devised, The Magician's Assistant, was a head-on encounter with a variety of words designed to have immediate image-appeal. I gave participants a workshop sheet on which were written a number of words relating to magic shows. I used very few abstracts, and those there were did the same job as the concrete words in flashing up instant pictures – 'conjure', 'doves', 'enchant', 'gloves', 'wand' – all of which, I hoped, would quickly jog participants' imaginations. I thought that most people in the group would be familiar with the concept of magic shows in some way or other, having watched them on television, having experienced them at celebrations, such as birthday parties, or having seen them live. I asked participants to write poems which included all or some of the words on the sheet. Although I had put the exercise together, its basis lay in the tried and tested notion of using connected images to provoke word and thought association and bring forward experiences, recollections and memories.

It's important to say at this point that the exercise followed one in which I'd asked participants to work within formal boundaries: that is, they worked within stanzas of (ideally) the same length. Here, these constraints had been taken away. This was deliberate: I wanted to see how participants felt about working freely with words, making their own forms and patterns. With the conceptual/perceptual barriers of structure removed, I thought it would be interesting to see if participants felt able to enjoy their creativity more fully and directly or, conversely, that some sort of safety net had been removed. The exercise was timed (15 minutes), after which we had a (voluntary) read-back and a discussion.

The exercise ended in the collective hush that comes before people start owning up to what's been written. One participant, Mark, was adamant that his work wasn't worthy, and made apologies before reading out a short, incisive and provocative poem that generated far more discussion/argument than its somewhat mystified creator had envisaged. He was both gratified and, I think, reassured by the honesty and sincerity with which his poem was treated and discussed. His reaction reinforced for me the importance of being aware of the complexity (and potential fragility) of every participant, even the most confident-seeming. After all, it wasn't only the creative unknown that participants were dealing with, but their own hidden psychologies and those of other participants.

The psychological and emotional complexity of individuals – both in terms of how they approached a creative task and how they presented the results to others – were made more apparent by the number of issues the exercise threw up. The first was the intensity of memory, both real and imagined. Another participant, Rachel, recalled the theatre and the stage where she had first seen a magic act; her act of remembering caused further acts of remembering within other participants. For me, the idea of a magic act, with its evanescent glamour, represented the sense of beauty fading. Helen subverted/inverted the exercise by developing a refusal to write *with* the words; instead she wrote against them, pulling them off the stage and into a love made all the stronger because it refused enchantment but faced the ordinary and still found wonder in it.

Another issue related to the fundamentals of personal development by highlighting how this can be hindered by the past and, crucially, by a failure of expectation or by expectation itself. Mark, who fretted over showing his work to the group; Rachel, who apologised before reading out her work; Lynne, who read apologetically: all demonstrated how circum-scribing expectation can be. Failure of expectation extended into the idea/desirability of being enchanted in some way – with life, with a person, with an idea – and the difficulties that arise when this belief/ aspiration is lost or suppressed.

From this came the importance of regeneration – emotional and spiritual. We examined the transforming element/transforming process of magic with a good deal of honest, sometimes cynical, often hopeful, discussion. We agreed that the concept of magic translated/extended into the idea of magic/hope in participants' lives, and looked at the ways in which it could be lost without someone necessarily being aware of it. The exercise itself seemed to stand for a good deal more than its face value; poetry is a useful tool for decanting emotions, issues, problems and experiences into something ostensibly less threatening. Somewhat cont-rarily, its perceived lack of directness (expressed through a medium, through metaphor, symbol, persona) enabled people to be more direct by proxy.

At the end of the discussion, I asked participants how they felt about the lack of formal structure. Some felt it enabled them to write more freely; others felt inhibited by it. In exploring why they felt this way, the latter group seemed (broadly) to feel that they were denied a point of reference from which to work. This kind of self-knowledge/self-examination – viewed as a luxury, or unnecessary, or discomfiting, depending on the individual – invariably extends out from poetry and into personal lives and development.

The theme of the workshop was Magic Words. In general, words are utilitarian, everyday tools which have nothing particularly remarkable about them – except, of course, that they enable us to communicate. But usually in a constrained way. We tend to use them to rein in our feelings, not to set them free. By engaging with the heightened sense of language that poetry demands (Seamus Heaney's 'language in orbit'), and by – for 15 or so minutes – entering a world of words, we disarmed for a little time at least this sense of constraint. This in turn enabled us to step down into group discussion and bring to it the same sense of transformation that made us move our pens across the paper in the first place. It is then, perhaps, that a different kind of honesty – deeper, more personal – begins to work, no matter how briefly. It's a process – not always comfortable – that is essential to understanding ourselves and, in doing so, developing our lives.

Magic

This is real
not some hocus pocus

Life isn't a stage
I don't care
whether the audience
claps or boos
or leaves
well before the interval

One other's enough

It wasn't the moon
on a midnight sea
that enchanted me

No one said abracadabra
or waved a wand

You didn't appear in a spotlight
I have no need of amulets
My spells are unbound

When I look closely
at, say, a rabbit
with its red-rimmed pink eyes
and nose in perpetual motion

or examine the velvety depths
of an empty hat

I am not resisting the magic
but just being –
unenchanted

here
now
in the perfect wonder
of you
in an imperfect world.

The Magician's Assistant

They have itched
a thousand tricks,
these tights,
furred with the rub
of her thighs,
their golden seams
now withering.

It has shone
a thousand stars,
this bodice,
a thousand eyes
a thousand hands
dealing magic
to curtains and flats.

They have framed
a thousand *presto* moments,

these gloves,
dazzling the pit
with their abracadabras.
No movement now,
scarlet and still.

If she could
she'd enchant herself again.

For the stage,
for the flowers and the doves,
for the amulet of hands clapping.

Acrostics   *Larry Butler*

ACROSTICS

CROSTICS

ROSTICS

OSTICS

STICS

TICS

ICS

CS

S

I use acrostics in many of the groups I facilitate. I find them to be good starters for folk who are new to poetry and, even in a group with mixed experience, they can be a good leveller. Most often a keyword is written vertically down the left margin. More difficult is a diagonal word across the middle of the text. The keyword could be the name of a person, an emotion, a colour, a theme, a place – it depends on what you want to create. You can usually achieve a satisfying result within a few minutes.

In late September I was part of a team leading a four-day residential training course: 'The Healing Power of Words – The Hurtful Power of Words'. We began the first evening with acrostic flash cards – our names written bold and bright and big vertically along the left margin using thick felt tips. After each letter, we wrote an expectation, hope or fear about the forthcoming workshops. One of my co-facilitators, Helen Boden, wrote:

> Hoping the self/other balance will be in balance
> Entering a retreat space
> Leaving time for things to just happen
> Exiting urban issues and concerns
> Nurturing what needs to be nurtured

Helen also did a follow-up by adding a response to each line when she returned home:

> Hoping the self/other balance will be in balance – more than I could have
>
>> hoped, if hard won
>
> Entering a retreat space – without withdrawing
>
> Leaving time for things to just happen – and not spending time monitoring
>
>> this constantly, but not slowing in body as much as I might
>
> Exiting urban issues and concerns – experiencing Autumn in the middle of
>
>> the nation, at the foot of the hill, in trees of birdsong
>
> Nurturing what needs to be nurtured – without thinking too hard what that
>
>> was; feeling nurtured and whole even when concerned about my health, and without needing to mention it: held in a safe space

One participant couldn't arrive until Day Two so we used the flash cards as a quick introduction.

AlphaPoems   *Kathleen Adams*

It was a sweltering day in late July. The air conditioning was malfunctioning, and my group room on the top floor of a 100-year-old psychiatric hospital was like a sauna. The adult unit was filled to capacity, and every one of the 18 patients came to journal therapy group that afternoon.

'It's too hot to write!' the patients complained as they poured in and filled every available chair, couch and floor pillow. 'We want to do something fun!'

'How about poetry?' I said. They groaned.

I turned to the whiteboard and wrote the alphabet, A to Z, vertically from top to bottom. 'Let's write a poem in which every line starts with the next letter of the alphabet,' I suggested. 'I'll start.' I wrote a title at the top of the board – 'An AlphaPoem on AlphaPoems' – and continued:

> Anticipate a
> Blossoming of
> Creative
> Delight!

'What's next?' I said. 'Who's got the next line or two?'

Silence.

> Easy, really, once you
> Find the rhythm and the pace

I continued. 'Who's got the G line?'

Sarah raised her hand tentatively. 'How about –

> Gather up the thoughts you
> Hold secret in your heart.

'Hey, that's two lines!'

Michael continued:

> Imagine them
> Just drifting out, a
> Kaleidoscope of
> Letters
> Making words.

Another voice chimed in a line. And another. Soon, with some minor editing and rearranging, we had finished the poem:

> No 'rules' to follow (except the
> Obvious one
> Perhaps you'll find a poet inside?
> Quite likely!

Re-read your AlphaPoems – you'll find them
Startlingly
True – an
Unusual way to give
Voice to the
Wails, whimpers, wonderings, whys, wins.
eXhilarating feeling to find
You've reached the
Zenith of the poem!

I looked around the room at 18 damp and flushed faces, all filled with the unmistakable light of creative engagement. 'Shall we do another?' I asked. They nodded.

'This time, I want you to write your own AlphaPoems,' I said. 'Write about something it's hard for you to talk about in therapy. Start by writing the alphabet down the side of your page, just like I did on the board. You've got ten minutes. Ready – set – go!'

Heads bowed, pens scratched. Ten minutes later, they began sharing their poems with each other. To their own (and, I admit, my own) astonishment, every one was a singular gem, an outpouring of raw, aching, honest, haunting stories.

Anxiety flows
Beneath my brow.
Creeps in muttering of
Doom and despair…

'Anger is
Best kept
Calm and collected.'
Dead I became because of this
Example…

A child once loved, and then
Betrayed.
Could it have been real?
Defenceless, innocent,
Every harsh word ever spoken
Feels like the lash of a whip…

Anorexia is lovely, as is
Bulimia, too. Just
Can't seem to get it right.
Death is near, and yet so far...

AlphaPoems have become a staple in my toolbox of journal therapy techniques. They are closely related to the simple poetic device of 'acrostics' explained earlier by Larry Butler.

The AlphaPoem format blends nicely with acrostic poems. It is very effective to take a therapeutic issue, such as 'substance abuse', or a therapeutic goal, such as 'making good choices', or even a generalised check-in, such as 'what's going on?', and use it as both the theme and the structure of the poem.

One of the primary differences between acrostics and AlphaPoems is continuity. In acrostics, the lines tend to be stand-alone, each one responding to the core theme (words or phrases that describe or identify 'Cathy'), but independent from each other. In an AlphaPoem, the lines flow into each other in a way that does feel poetic. In fact, it is often the case that when AlphaPoems are read aloud, the alphabetical structure falls away and what is left is a piece of writing that can credibly be called a poem.

The inevitable question that evolves at this stage is, 'But isn't it the case that the ones who write good AlphaPoems are just naturally good writers?' With my standard caveat in place (I think that *all* writing that comes from an authentic place within is 'good' writing), I will say that one of the most startling, surprising and consistent qualities of AlphaPoems written for therapeutic purposes is that it is precisely the writers in the group who are *least* developed, or least confident of their writing, who seem to have the greatest success with this form. Why is this? I cannot say with certainty, but I have a couple of ideas.

First, the patients and clients who come to us for journal therapy often have deeply embedded writing wounds. Some have internalised messages from primary or secondary school that they are poor writers, because assignments came back awash in red ink. Some have experienced ridicule for what they said, or how they said it, or how it looked on the page. Some grew up in families where reading and writing were not prized. Some wrote adolescent diaries or journals that were read without permission. They subsequently have a difficult time trusting that they can write about their innermost experiences without humiliation or punishment.

For these 'wounded writers' the sing-song structure of the alphabet may propel them back to their earliest relationship with spoken and written language, to a time before there were rules and impositions. They may find the form so comforting, so irresistibly familiar, that they plunge eagerly into the 'ABCs' and find themselves easily diving below the surface of years of conditioned response.

Second, after witnessing hundreds of AlphaPoems, I believe there may be a component to the structure that corresponds to object relations theory (a psychoanalytic theory which assumes that the primary human drive is a need for satisfying relationships with others and that the ability to form relationships is affected by early childhood experiences). There the next letter sits – known, fixed, constant, stable, sure. That allows exploration, a wild dive into the unknown, going out beyond the familiar, before returning to the safety of the next line's start.

Patients and clients – particularly those who do not think of themselves as successful writers – report that the poems 'write themselves', that they 'do not have to think' and that the next words 'simply appear'. When they read their AlphaPoems back, they often remark that they are deeply impressed by how 'true' they seem, by which they often mean that there is an accurate emotional resonance, or the emergence of an authentic voice. It thus appears that unconscious material is surfacing in a way that feels nonthreatening, useful, valid and even exciting.

Additionally, the self-esteem and shifted self-concept generated by an AlphaPoem is deeply gratifying for all concerned. It is delightful to witness a previously struggling patient or client begging to read out loud and beaming at the genuine admiration of their peers.

As our earliest AlphaPoem prophesied, there are 'no rules to follow, except the / obvious one' of starting the next line with the next letter. Even so, it is perfectly Xceptable to use Xceptions for Xtra hard letters. I encourage phonetic spellings, creative hyphenations and any other adaptations that will make the process flow. I came into my group room one day to find that some enterprising soul had made a poster filled with Z words from the dictionary.

More accomplished poets/writers – those who write easily and who have a sense of confidence about their writing – often report being 'bored' or 'constrained' by what they experience as the trivial or unnecessary structure of AlphaPoems. But for clients or patients who struggle, try an AlphaPoem. *Perhaps they'll find a poet inside?*

Group Poem: The Making of a Group   *Cheryl Moskowitz*

The effect of the group is a humanisation of the subject through the establishment of social bonds. (Rowan and Harper 1999, p.172)

When a group of people comes together and the members join their efforts into a collective act it never fails to move me. I find the sight of a congregation singing or praying together, demonstrators marching, chanting or joining together at a mass rally, or even a group of children simply gathered together for a school assembly profoundly stirring. My being moved has nothing at all to do with the content or quality of the activity or even my own connection or belief in it, simply the fact that many people are doing it together. It is the togetherness that moves me even though I know that the bond I might be witnessing between these fellow beings on these occasions is usually transitory and temporary. What is often missing from these gatherings is the creative impulse, the exchange of ideas, the gift of thought, heart and mind.

When I am given the opportunity to come as a writing facilitator into new groups of people to which I will often be a stranger, I make it my priority to have a collective moment, a point of coming together and bonding as early as possible in the life of the group. But in doing this I want to do more than effect a choir of voices singing the same hymn or an army acting on instruction in unison. I want to facilitate a collective moment where everyone feels an absolute sense of belonging and connection to one another and knows, absolutely, that the moment could not have happened without each one of them being present and participating. This is the thinking behind the 'group poem' that, more often than not, I do as one of the first exercises when beginning work with any new group. Cohesion, mutual appreciation and belonging feel like important prerequisites for further creative work.

The group poem should mark something that is relevant and important to everyone within the group and so the inspiration for it, its conception and construction should come out of a shared experience by the group. The more immediate, the better. The experience need not be huge, it can simply be about sharing the same space, being together in the same room and noticing, individually and collectively, what is found there.

If there is a different space which the group can easily enter – simply to walk, stand, listen, observe – then for novelty value or for reasons of freshness I might suggest doing that. A class of children can, for example, be taken out into their school playground at a time when it is not playtime (something I did recently to begin a story-writing project with eight classes of six- and seven-year-olds); a group of patients at a hospital can be taken into the hospital grounds or even onto a corridor or part of the hospital they don't often see. A group attending a workshop in a day centre or library can be invited to look out of a window together to see what they notice. People who have been meeting for some time in the same room can be invited to look closely at the floor or ceiling which they might not have bothered to look closely at before despite – or because of – the familiarity of the setting. If time and conditions allow, a group walk or journey to and from a designated spot can be very inspiring (I have taken groups into parks, gardens, through graveyards, to chapels and other places of worship and to the sites of old buildings).

During this time of journey or close observation (it could be five minutes, or in the case of a walk perhaps more like half an hour) pens and paper are provided and participants are invited to write; if they are too young or are unable to write themselves, I can be their scribe. At two or three points over the time I encourage people to stop, stand still and take time to register what they are seeing, hearing or feeling at that moment. I ask each individual to write down (or tell me so that I can write it down) what they have noticed. Ideally over the course of the journey/observation time everyone will have expressed themselves through a range of senses. The writing down can be in the form of single words, phrases or whole sentences.

Once back on home ground each person separates the words, phrases or sentences they have written by tearing or cutting them into strips. If there are many thoughts and ideas which have been generated I might ask each person to select three that they like the best from those they have written. Perhaps they will like what they have written because of the way it looks when written down, or for the way it sounds when it is said; because of what it means, what it expresses or what it reminds them of; or maybe simply because it feels like the best word or sentence they have written.

Inviting the group into a circle I collect all the strips together and read out what is written on each, one by one, to the group, placing them face up in the centre of the circle (on a table or on the floor where everyone can see them) as I do so. Once all strips have been read and are visible I ask the group to select one as a starting point for the poem (I would always take the first suggestion unless a strong consensus determines another one be used).

The poem is formed directly from what has been written on those strips of paper, ordered collectively by the group. The process is done visibly by moving the strips of paper around in the manner of cutting and pasting on a computer screen. After the first line of the poem has been decided – say it is a strip which reads 'I can see the sky' – then the group is invited to choose from the strips available a second line to follow the first and so on and so on.

Sometimes there is a theme or an obvious progression through the images or words provided which the group members will find for themselves. Sometimes they will be operating more poetically or aesthetically in their choice of ordering. If they are in a group which has difficulty cooperating in its choices they can be instructed to take turns in making the choice of the next line. It matters little whether there is an obvious logic to the line sequence or not. In poetry we will always find our own logic. The important thing is to read the lines aloud to the group as they begin to be linked together and assigned an order. They will hear the poem developing and be encouraged by its strange and unique beauty, and proud of their own individual contributions within it. Once all the strips are placed in their decided order I usually write the poem in full and offer to make copies for each member of the group to keep and remember.

To have a line that you have written chosen by someone else as the perfect line to go next in the formation of the poem is a wonderful and satisfying feeling. To see a line or a word that you were secretly worried others would find bland come alive in the context of the other lines which have been written is reassuring and exhilarating. To hear a poem emerge, even one which might sound odd and perhaps mysterious or even inscrutable to others not part of its making, is a deeply affirming and binding experience for a group. To have achieved this one moment of togetherness and shared pride in what they have produced is perhaps the best investment in all the group's moments to follow.

Telling Tales: Script Conference and Storytelling Exercise
Kate D'Lima

In an East London tower block a group of 12 women who were experiencing domestic violence came together for a creative writing session. One room was used for a crèche and women found it hard to separate themselves from their children. An Asian mother joined the group late and described how she had to prise tiny fingers from the hem of her coat. For around half this group, English was not their first language; other women were nervous about literacy, while some were very accomplished in written English. Despite this, they had responded positively to a three-hour creative writing session organised by a women's refuge which I had been asked to teach.

Thinking about creative writing, with its genesis in storytelling, the solution to these mixed abilities became clear. A script conference and storytelling exercise would help this group bond, since some had never met before, and would make the most of wide cultural experience. Script conferencing is a method used by a group to write episodes for television soaps and sitcoms and I borrowed some of these techniques. The story-telling angle solved the literacy and language problem, since it required only three women to write and they had to volunteer to do this. Everyone else was given strong participatory roles.

This exercise resulted in one of the most valuable sessions I have taught and proved that people do not physically have to write to participate in a creative activity. Also, it offered new ways of seeing life problems and brought some sensitive issues into a supportive environment.

Since storytelling was the theme, I devised a lesson plan that had a strong beginning, middle and end. I began with a session where all 12 women told a true story. Next, we had break-out sessions where three groups of four people formed script-conference teams to turn one of the stories told earlier into a storytelling presentation. Finally, the entire group reassembled to present and discuss the three finished stories.

In the first hour we had an ice-breaker session designed to get people talking to one another before devising ground rules such as confidentiality and feedback techniques. Each participant then told a true story about themselves or a woman family member such as their mother, sister or grandmother. The stories were varied and exotic – about the chance meetings of their parents, family secrets or escape from war-torn countries. One woman chose to tell a personal story of domestic violence and her midnight exodus with two small children from the family home. We sat like infants in rapt absorption.

After each story we gave brief feedback and talked about some of the techniques each storyteller used, such as suspense and delay, third person or first person narration, narrative voice, openings and resolution, to help introduce techniques they would use later. The group then divided into three by identifying three volunteer scribes who could catch the essence of the story as it developed. The rest of the women then followed a scribe into three separate rooms to plan their presentation. Each group had a flip chart, marker pens and a list of tasks. They had to choose a true story told earlier by a member of their group, appoint a storyteller and all contribute to turn the story into a piece of fiction which would take around five minutes to tell.

I visited each of the three groups and observed the script conferences in action. Attention rarely wandered and all women were confident and animated. They quickly came to a decision about which story to choose and I was surprised, maybe a little nervous, to realise that the real-life story of domestic violence was among those to have been chosen.

The presentations in the final session were fit for performance. A story of love and betrayal in a faraway land was given new fictional dimensions by group imaginations; a humorous tale of a family secret could have been given to a soap opera; but the story of domestic violence was inspirational. The group decided to transpose the true characters into farmyard animals and present it as a story for children. It can be summarised as follows:

> In a cold, damp farmhouse a family of kittens were held hostage
> by a cockerel who kept them awake crowing angrily every night.
> An old sheepdog, an owl and some geese got together and made
> a plan. On one of the blackest nights of the year, the cat tied
> orange bale-twine around her kittens' necks. The dog distracted
> the cockerel by barking and chasing it, whilst the geese held the
> twine in their beaks and led the family of kittens to the safety of
> a new barn under the guidance of the owl who hooted above.

The story encouraged open discussion about domestic violence and the woman whose story it was decided to tell this tale to her children. Other women felt it was good to transpose a personal story into a tale such as this, as a way of getting distance from an experience and new insight into a life problem. They felt the solution to violence within the family was more obvious when animals were concerned and that their children might find it easier to hear a tale such as this. There was also talk about how one can become isolated by a sense of shame associated with domestic violence and how this session helped break those barriers.

I have taught many creative writing courses to diverse groups in health settings, including a hospice, a drug and alcohol group and a mental health group. Since I am not a therapist, I teach writing as an art form. My research concerns the potential of creative writing to enable new ways of seeing and this session stands out as achieving those new perspectives.

CHAPTER 2

Writing about Place

Edited by Victoria Field

Places – real and imaginary, literal and metaphorical – are a useful and open-ended theme for many kinds of therapeutic writing. We often use place as a metaphor for more general feelings about our lives; the question 'Where are you at?' substituting for the more global 'How are you?' We talk about feeling 'at home' or 'all at sea' in certain situations or with certain people. This entire introduction is peppered with idioms referring to place that are so embedded in the language that we barely notice them.

Thinking about a childhood haunt, the specifics of our working environment or a favourite holiday destination can immediately evoke details that illuminate our current emotional landscape. A warm-up activity I often use is to ask whether people would rather be a kitchen or a bathroom. This tends to divide a group into clear halves, each arguing passionately for their choice. It is not the rooms themselves, of course, but the qualities deemed important that are often revealing.

There are numerous writing activities that can tap into this potent source of personal insights. They can be divided into four categories:

1. Writing about a real, remembered place
This is simply asking people to write about a place – either one that they know now or one from the past. A popular suggestion refers to a near-universal place: writing from the phrase 'In my mother's kitchen…', and, for those who may not have been brought up by their mother, their imagined mother's kitchen, can lead to powerful writing. Some groups may be daunted by writing continuous prose, in which case it is possible to use an opening phrase (sometimes called a 'sentence stem') to make a list poem – the work can be done either individually or orally with the facilitator 'scribing' the group poem. In *Writing for Self-Discovery*, Myra Schneider and John Killick (1998) suggest simply imagining a familiar room and making

up a series of sentences each opening with the three words 'the room where...'.

An alternative to beginning with the place itself would be for participants to identify, say, an emotion or a relationship and then write about the place which they associate with it. An exercise in 'show, not tell' might be to demonstrate the nature of the emotion or the relationship through the description of the place rather than by describing the emotion directly.

For example, people can be invited to recall places where they felt safe and secure as children and, conversely, places where they might have felt a sense of freedom and exhilaration. The balance and tension between challenge and security is often of concern in personal development and reflecting on places associated with each can be helpful. Caution, though, should be exercised in inviting writing about places where there was a real sense of danger, although, in an established therapeutic relationship, a client might value being able to write, perhaps obliquely at first, about a frightening space.

In the exercise in this chapter, I Know My Place, I describe participating in a workshop led by Angela Stoner in which participants wrote about a variety of real and imagined places.

2. A workshop based on visiting a real place

One of the objectives of many therapeutic writing workshops is to provide a space in which people are able to be fully 'in the moment'. One way of achieving this sense of being totally present is to work directly in or with a stimulating environment. Places of natural beauty are an obvious choice as engaging with nature *per se* has healing qualities that can be enhanced by close observation and writing. When I lead workshops on personal development holidays in southern France, or at the annual Resurgence summer camp (a forum for deep ecology), I begin by inviting people to walk silently through the fields, woods and gardens, simply writing down what they notice through all their senses – whether single words or complex descriptions. When these are read back 'Quaker-style', without commentary, the effect is of creating a multi-sensory portrait of an environment in which repetitions and echoes complement individual voices in such a way that a group of strangers immediately feels part of something larger.

In this chapter, Judy Clinton vividly describes how being by the sea facilitated a workshop in which people wrote 'from the *depths* of their beings' (my italics) and, in Riverlines, Linda Goodwin contrasts the experience of leading workshops in clinical, multi-use spaces with being able to see autumn sun sparkling on water.

An inspiring built environment, such as a castle, stately home or a quiet village (especially if it has a writer-friendly café), is especially useful in generating stories. One technique is to suggest writing about a personal experience but setting the action in the current environment in a specific historical period. The workshop can be developed further by experimenting with first and third person writing or, Orlando-style, changing the gender of the protagonist.

Miriam Halahmy here describes a writing workshop at Kenwood House on the edge of Hampstead Heath, where nature, the city and outdoor sculptures combine to offer both inspiration and serenity.

3. Place as metaphor

Describing an aspect of one's life – such as a significant relationship, a team at work, home life – as if it were, for example, a garden can be a playful way of engaging with both its valued and disliked characteristics. In 2004, convenors of Lapidus local groups did this exercise to develop a vision of how they wanted their groups to be – the resulting gardens had bridges and fountains, flower beds and weedy areas, hammocks and gates – all of which lent themselves to more metaphorical explorations of what an organisation can be.

This kind of writing works best when the metaphor is capable of encompassing complexity and change – using a garden or a fictitious country or a landscape can enable the writer to describe actual or desired changes over time.

In Chapter 1, page 37, I described a workshop warm-up exercise in which participants introduce themselves as if they are specific places – the intention being that by exploring a metaphor orally, there is more room for spontaneity and an instinctive engagement with the metaphor.

4. Guided imagery

This technique involves a facilitator taking people to different places in their imagination, usually after a series of breathing and relaxation exercises. Some guided imagery exercises follow a narrative pattern such as a 'quest'; others invoke different personae, such as our inner child, anima or animus; and yet others focus on a specific place. This process is sometimes described as a kind of conscious dreaming as the relaxed state often allows unexpected images to come into consciousness. Not only can our, often unexpected, choice of imagery reveal unconscious concerns and processes, but it can clarify possible alternative courses of action. A wealth of such exercises is described in Dina Glouberman's (1995) book *Life Choices, Life Changes: Develop Your Personal Vision with Imagework*, all of which can be adapted for writing.

In this chapter Susan Kersley describes a beautifully simple guided visualisation in which professionals imagine the work space of a colleague, real or imagined, whom they consider outstanding; while Myra Schneider offers a selection of what she calls 'image explorations' and suggests that the implicit permission to use a mixture of fantasy, reality and metaphor is especially helpful for people writing about painful experiences.

I Know My Place   *Victoria Field*

It is a Wednesday morning in November 2004 and a group of us gather at 'Far West', a beautiful private home and writing centre in a very old street. We are eight women and one man seated around a granite table in the alcove of the kitchen. Light is pouring in, coffee and tea are being poured out and there are, of course, generous plates of biscuits. This is a Hobnob – a peer meeting where Lapidus members facilitate a therapeutic writing workshop for other members. Today, Angela Stoner is offering a three-hour session and, whilst six of us know each other well, and regularly facilitate our own workshops, there are two new-comers: members of Angela's weekly writing group for women who are new to writing as well as to Lapidus. Angela introduces the theme – I Know My Place – and invites us to write freely for six minutes in the knowledge that what we write will not be read aloud. Soon, the somewhat fractured atmosphere of arriving, getting seated, having coffee and so on coalesces into one of focus and the sound of pen on paper. At the end of six minutes, there are sighs, yawns and stretching – and for most of us, the familiar experience of the writing almost 'writing itself' has moved us from concern with the outer world to deep engagement with the inner world. There are smiles as we relax into the workshop.

For the next piece of writing, Angela invites us to write about a place from our childhood: a den or hiding place. Here, I find I am challenged. Somehow, the phrase 'I Know My Place' takes on sinister overtones. There is the hint of the martyr speaking and ideas of limitation. I am suddenly unsure about the group. I want to write from a deep place but I also fear exposing myself. The childhood place that I think of is a patch of woodland where I and a group of friends attempted to make a camp – nothing sinister happened there but it has taken on an iconic quality of darkness associated with other incidents in childhood. I decide to honour the process and to write whatever comes to mind but to reserve for myself the right not to share it. The only way I am able to write at all is by hurling myself at the subject matter. The following is the stream of consciousness that emerged:

> The place, the place, the place
> A childhood den? Not really
> The rooks, the rooks, the rooks
> The non-place, the deep woods
> The not-safe place, the anemones, dead
> The dense leaf-mould, the little fire
> The faceless friends, the dusk, the high trees
> The wheeling rooks, the sharp twigs and brambles
> The deepening wood, the smouldering fire
> The damp smoke, the being with them
> The children with forgotten names
> The black sound of the birds, the absent sun
> No den at all, just branches, bracken, brittle days
> A note under a stone, the faces I no longer know
> The paper wet and lost, the words unread
> The rooks above who simply won't
> Shut the fuck up.

I then had the sense of surprise that such freewriting often engenders. I was astonished that, whilst I remembered the woods clearly, I was unable to name any of my childhood playmates of the time. I also shocked myself by the vehemence of the end of what I wrote. I resolved not to share it.

Angela then suggested going deeper into a sensory exploration of the place. I wrote a 'list poem' about woods – balancing the earlier piece by thinking of woodlands that I love. An extract reads:

The wet scent of walking
The sweet scent of breathing
The smiling scent of growing
The wild scent of life longing for itself…

I knew as I wrote that I was playing safe, that the writing had no energy or power behind it and I was selling the process short.

Finally, Angela then suggested summarising our writing in 50 words. I wrote:

> Sometimes, the girl went with her friends to a copse on the outside of the village where she lived. It was a scruffy patch of trees, what kind she can't remember, with a large rookery. The children made a fire but, with everything being so damp, it didn't take.

We were then invited to share our writing. As the others read aloud, I was reminded of the power of the sharing stage of therapeutic writing. Through their words, we were taken on journeys to precisely imagined and conjured worlds. When Philip, the only man present, read his piece, it set up echoes with my own and the pleasure of the synchronicity that often happens in workshops encouraged me to share. I also felt that I wanted to express aloud the angry phrase I had written – and certainly there was a feeling of catharsis in doing so, helped by laughter from some of the others.

Angela pointed out the use of the third person in my final piece – something she had observed before in my writing – but which was quite unconscious. In these workshops the quality of the listening is paramount but often a factual observation or reflection can be very helpful to participants.

Angela then presented us with three published poems demonstrating a clear engagement with place which opened the discussion into other books and poems that had encouraged us to look at place.

Finally to close the workshop, Angela invited us to write about an idealised place, a perfect place. My first piece of flow writing had reflected uncertainties and feelings of not belonging. This last piece enabled me to see the positive side of change and uncertainty but, unlike the middle piece of writing on a childhood place, it felt authentic and not Pollyanna-ish. It also enabled me to neutralise some of the negative associations I had with 'I Know My Place' and for me to re-hear it as an affirming, clear statement.

Part of the piece reads:

> I know my place as an open road
> I am never as light and free as when my boots
> are on a path from somewhere to somewhere else
>
> I know my place as the buzz of the departure lounge
> the plane on time, the suitcase checked
> the thought of different smelling air at the other end
>
> I know my place as an unwalked street
> in a sunny city where something will happen
> in a language I don't understand...

This was an extremely productive workshop for me. The focus on place helped me to reframe my experience of changes in my life from simply uncertain to the excitement of going on a journey. The unexpected insights and emotional reactions to the writing about childhood places gave me food for thought and material for further exploration. But, not least, the symbolic sharing of our writing in a safe space threw new and unpredictable shafts of light on to one another's insights and gave us all new ways of looking at our own and others' places.

A Workshop with the Theme of the Sea   *Judy Clinton*

In June 2004 I facilitated a weekend workshop within a spiritual comm-unity by the sea who opened their doors to interested people for retreats and workshops. I had spent a time with this community myself and it was through that connection that I had come to be working there. As they had a wide mailing list I was spared the effort of finding the participants, which was a great relief. The people who came were of different ages, sexes and backgrounds. Two people were disabled and many were bereaved for one reason or another. The workshop had been billed as a time for personal and spiritual reflection through the vehicle of spontaneous writing and empathetic sharing. Interestingly the subject of grief had not been mentioned, but given that I had myself been working through this condition for the previous three years, I may have psychically or unconsciously called people together with that concern. I have observed this phenomenon of attraction between facilitators and groups before and think it worthy of consideration.

The weather was spectacular that weekend and the scenery magnificent with views from our accommodation of piercing blue sky, sparkling horses on the sea and palm trees in the foreground. We could easily have been on the Mediterranean. Making use of our surroundings was the most obvious stimulation for our writing and sharing.

Before the workshop began I walked the beach for hours, absorbing the atmosphere and allowed the sea to 'speak' to me. It gave me the perfect opportunity to leave my home and work responsibilities behind and to move towards a more inward, contemplative condition. If I wasn't in a state of peace and serenity within myself then how could I hold such a space for the people who were coming to work with me? It reinforced my already held belief that holding such workshops is more about depth of presence than cleverly designed exercises. I was fortunate indeed to have this opportunity and reflected that this kind of pre-workshop centring had to be part of my future practice.

I collected pebbles from the beach and bunches of flowers to arrange in the centre of the room – it set the scene and brought the sea into the room for those unable to make their way to the beach themselves.

The first evening, when people were tired from the week and their journey, was slow and gentle of input. An experienced facilitator friend had advised 'Remember: less is more', and it proved to be so. It was a time for introductions. I spoke for a while about my own relationship to writing: how it had helped me personally and spiritually and how I was now passing on this powerful tool to others in many settings and for different kinds of people. Then each person spoke for a bit: sharing their names, where they had come from, what religious affiliation they had – if any – and what they hoped to gain from the weekend. We were a rich and varied group. We finished our time together by writing fast, non-stop for six minutes – a free-flow exercise designed to break the structured, rational, planned way in which most of us have been trained. This was a new experience for many people and they were all pleasantly surprised both by their capacity to do it and by what came out of them. It was a good point on which to rest, in silence, before the end of the day.

The following day, after some more spontaneous writing and another exercise (in which participants were asked to put the first word they thought of in the middle of the page and then draw lines from it to other associated words), we were ready to move on to writing of greater depth and duration. I stimulated this by offering the biblical text, 'Whatsoever

things are good…' We wrote for 20 minutes, locating ourselves outside or
in the buildings. Sharing followed, according to the rules of creative
listening: listening in receptive silence to all that was shared and then
contributing comments, if requested, of a constructive nature on the
content, not the form, of what a person had written. At every stage people
were in charge of their own process – they did not have to share, nor did
they have to receive feedback. In practice most people did.

The afternoon was programmed 'free time', although I did tell people
that we would be writing about the sea later and that they might like to
bring back things if they went to the beach. When we gathered together
again I played a tape of the sound of the sea for the benefit particularly of
those who had not been able to get to the beach. And then we wrote again
for 20 minutes. Sharing followed. We entered into what I can only describe
as a sacred space where people shared from the depth of their beings – of
their joys and their sorrows.

All of this was sparked by the subject of the sea and led to questions of
eternity and meaning. This poem was written by a man in the group who
later wrote, 'I think it is about grief and life and acceptance through the
medium of love.'

What Already Is by James Wilson

The sea with its endless shores around the world
Heaves and sighs, spuming white spray over dry land
Caressing smooth edges as it makes love
To its earth bride, dancing delicately, roughly
In the morning tide, shimmering in rock pools
On banks of pebbles shaped by a so-long-ago touch.
Sharp-eyed gulls cry above the water's low moan
As the sea embraces lonely shores, the birds circling
Like time itself, hungry for love to live a warm life in.
So many moods, twists and turns to take, to surrender
To each moment, each separate wave as it collapses
Sea-shapeless to create another wave, another shape
Effortlessly folding and unfolding, form without form
Light playing with dark, birth with death without end
Without beginning, without meaning, without trying
To make sense of what just is, what always shall be.

He also wrote that it was written 'under the duress of 20 minutes'! What remarkable work can come from a spontaneous approach and a time limit. His was not the only piece that was so moving and full of both personal and spiritual truth. Through a mixture of atmosphere, structure, mutual trust, opportunity and readiness to be open, people were able to share at great depth and with vulnerability; all aided by the sea.

Riverlines   *Linda Goodwin*

Rising slowly from the bench where he had been sitting in the sun, the Japanese gentleman walked tentatively over the rough ground towards 20 pairs of expectant eyes. Our cluster opened to admit him and re-formed in a circle around him. The open book was placed carefully in his hands; he looked at the page and hesitantly began to read the haiku. His voice was strangely high pitched and he faltered over some of the sounds even though he was reading his mother tongue. It was short and soon finished. He looked for reassurance from anyone and everyone surrounding him. His audience nodded and spoke words of gratitude. He moved out of the circle and disappeared.

As a writer in health care most of the workshops I facilitate are held in premises of varying degrees of suitability. They vary from rooms of multi-usage in which other clients are playing dominoes and making coffee, where the sizzle of the deep fat fryer brings everyone's attention towards the immediacy of the lunch break; to spaces where a flimsy display board separates writers from carnival Mas Band creators and computer-bound office staff. Add to these the clinical spaces provided within the hospital environs and adaptability becomes a prerequisite for this work.

However, a beautiful day in autumn saw a mixed group of writers gather at a causeway and watch the low sun sparkle on the shallow water. This was one of a series of gatherings that developed into a project entitled Riverlines in which visits were made to different river locations, images captured on film and poems written.

The assembled client group comprised members of a day centre, a poetry group, a carers' group, writers in health care and a photographer. The meeting place had been predetermined and information distributed to groups who might be interested in joining the party. Those who met on this brilliant morning were people who wrote poetry as a means to explore their feelings and channel their thoughts. All had attended groups run by writers in health care on the Isle of Wight; some were very experienced whilst others were just beginning.

Once assembled, our minds were soon enveloped in the magic of the location. The river tumbled over polished stones, splashing droplets into the air. Light shafted through overhanging branches and birds sang. Everyone absorbed the atmosphere, sharing observations and anecdotes. Local people stopped and chatted, adding to the stories already known, and a man from Japan sat on a seat nearby.

In a grassy space close to the water my colleague read a haiku to the group. The book she used displayed both the original verse and its translation side by side. I looked towards the Japanese gentleman and smiled; tentatively I asked him if he would mind reading the haiku to us in its original form. He was taken aback but agreed to my request. As we all stood listening to this stranger reading in his mother tongue the feeling of a unique coincidence crossed our minds and our focus sharpened.

Haiku is a useful form to use on location. It is concise and many thoughts can be honed into this succinct form, which consists of 17 syllables generally divided into three lines consisting of five syllables, followed by seven then another five. The first line contains a natural image; the second continues that image and adds movement; the third brings some truth to the whole. It is the nature of haiku that there is always an uplifting feeling in the third line.

Writing a haiku collaboratively as we then did gives the group feelings of security and exploration. All suggestions are considered and words chosen through consensus: words that conveyed the enchantment of the location and the sense of togetherness that was felt.

> Bones of the jetty
> stagger into blue water,
> searching for lost summers

We had met and wandered along beside the water sharing thoughts and silence for a couple of hours. We had listened to poems in English and Japanese and written a collaborative haiku; the photographer had captured the scene; the morning had been eventful and rewarding, and the location had given us lasting memories. Most of all we had been struck by the coincidence of a Japanese gentleman sharing and enriching the moment.

Inspiration and Serenity: A Workshop in the Outdoors
Miriam Halahmy

Kenwood House is an eighteenth-century mansion set in its own grounds
high above London on the edge of Hampstead Heath. When it was built
you could stand on the terrace and see the masts of tall ships sailing down
the Thames. It is a perfect place to write. The woods are a mist of bluebells
in spring and there are swans on the lake.

I therefore offered to run a workshop in June 2004 in the park for the
London Lapidus group. My plan was to include three outdoor sculptures,
the woods and lake, and finish with a panoramic view over London. I felt
sure that everyone would feel inspired to write in such a place.

Once the group had gathered we set off to a glade surrounded by giant
rhododendrons to the east of the house. In the centre of the glade is a tall
slender Barbara Hepworth sculpture, with a long opening down the centre.
The group settled down on the grass and I explained that the first activity
was for them to write about what they thought they could see through the
long opening in the centre of the sculpture. The writing which emerged
was deeply evocative and imaginative. Kate Thompson's poem began:

> Through the pinhole camera of the female form
> Shrouded in shreds of spiders' webs
> A suspension of dead fly dots against the
> Cerulean expansiveness of sky

Richard Wright imagined himself transported across the globe:

> Easter Island with its eye open
> Sideways ocular: not predacious

I had decided that we would read back work during our picnic midway
through the afternoon, so we walked along a path and through a gate onto
the heath, to the second sculpture. This piece provoked a lot of discussion
as it stood away from the path, in long rough grass, and appeared to have its
back to us. The writing which emerged reflected our strong and quite
controversial feelings about this lonely figure with its back to the world.
Was it rejecting us or longing to join us? Alison Clayburn reached out to
the figure in her writing:

> And here we have a sculpture (rough figure as if hewn) with its
> back turned to the path, but going around through the long

seeded grass, it's as if you meet it and see its twisted agony, the way its frame is pulled to one side, its long dejected arms stuck into unseen pockets. So then I am glad to be some company for him.

Sally Thompson's writing tried to enter both the minds of the passer by and the lonely figure:

> Those who pass you
> Engulfed by their own atrocities
> Mistake your sadness for indifference
> But you hold it
> This mourning for a lost understanding
> This denial of your life's blood
> And you cannot put it down

We walked on in reflective mood, re-entered the park and stopped by my favourite sculpture, a monumental Henry Moore, commanding a view over the great sweep of grass which leads up to the House. The piece consists of two figures and I suggested that we write a conversation, perhaps a lover's quarrel. Alison Clayburn entered into the spirit, as one figure says to another:

> I can only use these words because I have been incarnated in such a solid way, it has given me the power to speak – to speak out to you, to face you even though that projection is so close to me. It's as though I see it now for what it is – something given, not something you asked for... I love the power in your torso, I love the power in your back...

By this time we had been writing and walking for over an hour and so we decided to picnic under the trees near the lake. It was an opportunity to share food and our writings. It was also a chance to discuss the value of writing in such a setting. Leone Ridsdale commented on how she appreciated the opportunity to write in such a wide open space. This is reflected in a piece of writing she did after lunch:

View from the hill

> So there's London – it looks toy-townish below. I can see the Post Office Tower, sad since it closed that rotating restaurant – big and immobile. And then there's The Wheel – how it is lively. I cannot see it moving, but it is, I know – full of excited tourists

in its pods going up and coming down, a continuous fairground – playtime in front of serious Parliament, and far off left is the penis-shaped Swiss Re – taller than almost anything beside it, but much more organic. It could just be an extension of the wood.

Richard commented that he had picnicked on the heath 25 years earlier and was flooded with memories. 'People underrate nostalgia: its power to disturb. The day made me reflect on my 30 years in London. Many years, many emotions, so much done and undone.'

For the remainder of the afternoon we walked through the woods up to the top of the heath and some people continued writing. The group gathered, relaxed and refreshed, as we had a final read-back over tea in the walled garden café of the house.

Running a writing workshop in the outdoors provides the opportunity to take a group into a completely new environment and allow them to reflect on their own lives, in relation to new and different stimuli. I feel strongly that in relation to writing for personal development the group really benefited from such peaceful and beautiful surroundings. Kenwood is an oasis of country calm in a frenetic city and can provide the writer with an inner release which can release deep and often satisfying reflective writing.

A Corridor with Many Doors   *Susan Kersley*

In October 2004, I facilitated two workshops for doctors, as a life coach, writer and retired doctor, and took my first steps in using reflective writing as a tool during these.

The first time was with a group of 15 senior registrars, soon to be consultants in genito-urinary medicine in a city hospital. The title of my workshop was 'How to be an Outstanding Consultant' and it lasted two hours.

I offered the group some guided imagery: I asked them to close their eyes and imagine walking down a corridor with many doors, one of which had their name on it. I suggested they go inside that room and look around and be aware of how they felt in that room. Then to cross the corridor into a colleague's room (known or imaginary colleague) whom they regard as outstanding and notice what they liked about this person and their room. Then I brought the workshop participants back to our seminar room and asked them to write about the experience.

I didn't ask them to read their writing to the whole group or even to small groups, but instead to talk about what they noticed, first in small groups and then back to the big group.

There was plenty of positive feedback about this exercise including surprise from one about how her own room seemed like a prison. The preferable room in many cases was bright and sunny and they felt relaxed in it. Several participants referred to the 'bad room' and the 'good room'.

We talked in the group about what they could do to make the changes from how things are to how they would like them to be, and what would be the first step for them in this process. One doctor said she would start to swim regularly. Her first step was putting her swimming things in her car so she could stop at the pool on her way home.

Encouraged by this I did a similar guided imagery exercise a few days later with a group of senior family doctors in mid-Wales, all of whom were new GP principals. They were part of a supportive group which had met regularly over the past year (but had not met me before). The subject of this workshop was 'Looking after Yourself' and it lasted three hours, so this time I asked them to think about their own life and how they would like it to be. Again there was positive feedback from the majority of participants about using reflective writing as a tool to use for enjoying a better-balanced life. As a result, participants promised the group they would exercise more, go home from work earlier and do more to look after themselves more effectively.

Both groups of doctors were not used to either guided imagery or reflective writing so there were one or two who didn't like what they called the 'touchy feely' approach. They were expecting a formal lecture!

I feel encouraged by these two experiences and shall go on next time to specifically asking participants to read some of their writing to each other in small groups.

Image Explorations   *Myra Schneider*

Image explorations offer a framework in which the writer can make imaginative journeys using whatever mix of fantasy, reality and metaphor she/he chooses without feeling any pressure to label or focus directly on personal experience. The technique often offers a way of approaching material that is too painful to write about directly. Here are details of The Cave, an image exploration which I have found very potent:

1. Imagine you are by yourself in a cave (or write as she/he). There is only a little light and it is very quiet. Picture the cave's shape, its walls, ledges, crevices. Can you see water, stalagmites or stalactites? Think about some of these things: the ground underfoot, the temperature, the dimness, the smell. Write about what you can see, touch and smell. Include your feelings and maybe how you came to be in the cave.

2. You hear a sound or sounds which has or have a strong effect on you. Write about this.

3. You become aware of someone or something in the cave. Find a way of developing the piece.

(I suggest 8–12 minutes for each section.)

I thought up The Cave as an exercise for writers attending a residential course, 'Outer and Inner Landscapes'. At the time I was undergoing chemotherapy and I wasn't well enough to attend the course, but my exercise was set by another tutor with exciting results. I tried it out too with a small group at home and found it opened up surprising possibilities for myself as well as the participants. I've now used it a number of times and am always struck by the way it invites writers to travel within themselves, and also the many different kinds of cave they come up with.

The exercise was particularly successful at a one-off two-hour session with a group at a complementary treatment centre for cancer sufferers. The six women taking part had little or no experience of writing and they didn't know each other. Some had finished treatment recently, others were still undergoing treatment. They needed to talk and share the story of their illness and some mentioned other problems. I was very aware it was important to them that I too had been a cancer sufferer. Although they spoke easily one or two of them found it quite difficult to do an exercise which invited them to dump preoccupations, but they all enjoyed The Cave. I was impressed by the ways they found to write about healing. Here are extracts from pieces written by two members of the group:

> I am standing on a shingle beach in a cave in the Mendips. A clear pale blue lake ripples on the shore and at the far end of the cave disappears under a wall of rock...
>
> At first I am pleased to be alone and enjoy the feast of sensual pleasures; colours, reflections, sound and a pleasing chill that only touches me where my skin is bare.

Then I sense past inhabitants and a deep and ancient fear grips my belly. I hear the shingle scrape behind me and turn to see the form of a huge bear silhouetted against the light. At first I think it will attack me, but it looks into my eyes and then lumbers away across the cave floor up a previously unseen passage. (Heather Collins)

The cave feels cold and devoid of warm life. Its walls are hard and pitted with ridges. Protruding stacks reach up to meet the pointed rock fingers. I cannot see a path inviting me along my way... I hear a loud crash. My ears turn instinctively towards the source of the noise. The clues tell me it is a heavy object slicing through the surface of a pool of water... I gradually become aware of the wall on my left side. I begin to make out shapes in the rock face. I can see now its surface has a golden tinge. The loud crash has confronted the darkness. The falling rock has sucked behind it a tail of white from the sky outside. (Jane Carmichael)

The session made a strong impression on the group and afterwards they organised themselves to meet fortnightly to talk and try out the writing ideas in my book, *Writing My Way Through Cancer* (Schneider 2003).

Most of the workshops I run are for writers. However, I discovered early on as a writing tutor that many people attend creative writing groups because they feel a strong need to explore personal material. Here are outlines of two other image explorations which I have found worked well.

Crossing the Bridge

1. You are standing at the edge of a narrow bridge which has no rails. You want to cross to the other side but are worried about the dangerous drop below you. Describe the bridge, your surroundings, why you want to cross, how you feel.

2. You become aware of a person or people on the far bank. They are calling to you. Write about this and the effect on you.

3. Develop the piece of writing.

In the Wood

1. You have lost your way in a wood. There is no obvious way ahead. Describe your surroundings, the weather, how you came to be lost, how you are feeling.

2. You become aware of a clearing and are drawn to a creature, cottage or ruin in it. Write about this and the effect on you.

3. Do you find anyone in the clearing? Write what happens next.

Here is an extract from a piece written by Philippa Lawrence during a one-off six-hour workshop in Salisbury for Kickstart Poets.

> Smell of wet leaves, mulch from last autumn. I've never had a sense of direction so any way I take will probably be the wrong one; and how do I know I won't be worse off, further away from the road; emerge in a field with a bull in it. Countrymen carry guns for a reason, not just to poach game or rabbits. My father had a rifle when I was a little girl in Devon: said he'd shoot us all – my mother, grandmother and me – and as many Germans as he could before they got him, if they invaded. What I was trying to escape from at the pretty, thatched cottage would have been worse than being lost in a wood...

CHAPTER 3

Writing from Objects

Edited by Gillie Bolton

Using objects to help stimulate writing can lead people to dive into deep areas of memory and experience. Handling, sniffing, listening to, sometimes even tasting, objects takes people out of their brains and into their senses. Touch, smell, hearing, taste can have deep links into us; it is easy to become too reliant upon sight, and forget to pay attention to our other senses.

Focusing upon something outside and tangible can help shift writers' attention away from themselves and their immediate concerns. Paying attention to the thing and writing about it can feel fun, intriguing, a bit different. All this can loosen people up to write more freely. Yet what they write about is invariably, in one way or another, themselves and their pressing concerns. The object gives them an oblique focus. This, of course, is what so many of the exercises in *Writing Works* do in many different ways. The tangibility of objects, the way they make people use senses other than sight, can make them a powerful writing stimulus.

The objects used might be provided by the facilitator. Fiona Hamilton brought plasticine, Glynis Charlton an empty box, and Angela Stoner stones. They might be brought by the writers, as Angela Stoner's group brought their personal 'talismans' to write about, Geraldine Green's feathers and stones, and Fiona Hamilton's brought 'objects which were important to them'.

The objects might be miscellaneous or relate to each other thematically such as the feathers and stones. Objects might be brought into the place where the writing is to take place, or people might go out to find them, as when Geraldine Green took her group to the Roman museum. Or the group might find things in the environment of the workshop, as Helen Boden does. One workshop I have done many times involves asking the whole group to go out into the garden (when there's time, where there is a garden and when it's not raining), and find a very few things to experience with each one of their five senses. I remember a very touching poem about the taste of rose petals. This is a simple, yet superbly effective workshop.

Objects can stimulate memory pathways, possibly not explored for many years, or they can stimulate fruitful metaphorical connections.

Surprises can happen when using objects, as they can with any writing stimulus. These exercises can take people to their raw boundaries. Once, when I shook out my large and varied hat collection, inviting people to try them on, one woman instantly burst into tears. Her son had been a policeman; my collection includes a helmet. The whole group supported her. See also Robert Hamberger's thoughts in the exercise Feeling, Smelling, Hearing, Tasting Perhaps, But Not Seeing later in this chapter.

Singing Baked Bean Tins and Other Talismanic Objects
Angela Stoner

Talismans

Allowing an object to 'speak' and writing down what it 'says', 'communing' with objects as talismans, is a simple, effective exercise. I have participated in these exercises with any number of writing facilitators, including Gillie Bolton, Myra Schneider, Michael Laskey and Frances Wilson, and the exercise is a favourite of mine. I don't know who first thought of it as a writing exercise, but communing with objects in this way seems to be as old as humanity, and instinctive. Children readily speak to objects, and shamans use objects as a way to commune with the spiritual world. We seem to have a natural tendency to imbue objects with symbolic significance.

The first time I ever led a writing group I was naturally nervous, so spent ages planning and preparing material – lots of photocopies of Ted Hughes' writings, lots of structured writing activities, gathered from various sources. Yet I was woken up at 5 a.m. after a really strong dream in which my collection of stones shouted 'Listen to us!' As a result, I abandoned all my plans and just told the group to choose a stone, that it would 'speak to them' and that they were to write what they heard. I guided them through thinking about the senses, really handling and smelling the object, and asked them to write holding it in their non-writing hand. I gave them ten minutes for this exercise. The directness and immediacy of the writing was quite astonishing. It also appeared to break the ice of a new group by giving them a focus other than themselves.

People commented on how easy it was to write because it wasn't them but the stone who was talking. Somehow the stones helped open up a space in which the group could learn to trust each other and work together at a deep level. This group still meets regularly, five years after that first meeting.

I find that if there is time to be with an object for a long time, say an hour, just writing from it, you can enter something like a meditative state. I was once in a workshop led by Frances Wilson, and she asked us to just choose any object and write about it. It has been my experience that even the most mundane objects, teabags or loo paper, can yield deep insights. I remember writing a profound dialogue with a blackcurrent drink bottle at a workshop led by Gillie Bolton.

I recently advertised a series of workshops which I described as 'Writing for Connection'. Many of the women attending these workshops were going through harrowing/confusing life-change experiences – divorce, illness, nursing very ill partners, depression, etc. We met at a place called Chy Gwella (Cornish for House of Creativity and Healing). There was varied experience of writing among the group: one member had published books, two had attended other writing groups which I lead, and others had done little creative writing since leaving school. The initial course was for eight sessions altogether. Each one lasted three hours, and each time we focused on a different aspect, such as healing, strength or wisdom. At the beginning of the course, I asked each woman to find a talisman, and after a few weeks I asked them to bring their talismans to the workshop. I asked them to write down what their talisman had to say about their own inner strength.

This is what Elaine's bottle had to say:

> Small bottle from beach, what can you tell me about my sources of strength?

> Well, that you've kept them bottled up of course. That there's a lot more strength in you than you've ever allowed to come out, and now you're getting to that time in your life where, however battered and worn you're feeling, you need to take the cap off and let your strength, your inner strength, the courage of your convictions, the possibilities and potential of your personality, come pouring out – as a libation to yourself and to others, to friends and family. Otherwise you might as well take this bottle and chuck it back into the sea. Forget your ambitions and desires. Lock yourself all up again and soldier on miserably. But you know that you don't really want to do that. You know that it

would hurt more, having come this far, to turn back, and that you'd always regret it. So be positive – drink deep and live large!

There were a couple of women who'd forgotten to bring their talismans. I said that they could ask any object they had on them. Here is what Ali's nebuliser had to say:

> I am your lifeline to inspiration. I'm clear and transparent, yet provide a strong barrier against germs, pollution and evil. I am like your writing, enabling you to see clearly, protecting you against the emotional and psychic pollution in which you live.
>
> Deep breathing. Deep writing. Breath and words which reach right into your soul. Open your lungs as huge as you can. Let inspiration pour in. Let your soul expand. Listen. You can't breathe out until you've breathed in. That's inspiration. Wait. Look. Listen. Let your pen write and your thoughts follow.

And this is Janet's pendant which she had made in a jewellery class:

> When I went into the kiln and was seared by the heat
> My copper became green and purple
> Like hard crystal rock
>
> The copper wire and black enamel fused into me
> and coiled its strength into my surface and into my soul.
>
> I am strong, hardened in the fire
> with the age old green of the sea
> and the black and purple of the earth.
>
> There are more like me
> but we are all different,
> guarding our colours and strengths.

It is clear how each writer is able to understand and use metaphor. I think this illustrates how we are able to project onto objects aspects of ourselves which we cannot ordinarily recognise, or find difficult to acknowledge. By objectifying these aspects, and making them more concrete, we are somehow able to write straight from the subconscious. It literally objectifies our understanding of abstract aspects of self.

All of the above pieces were written in six minutes.

Other exercises with objects

Another exercise which I used with this group is a version of the consequences game which I call The Quest. People pass round unseen a piece of paper. The hero/ine is on the first line, who or what will hinder them is on the next, the quest or problem on the next, a magical object on the next, and finally an unexpected outcome of the successful quest is on the last line. I don't always ask people to write the actual quest. When people have the completed set, I give them 20 minutes to write up the plot as briefly as possible. Again, despite the hilarity of tone which often emerges, and the mundanity of some of the objects (I've had a rainbow toilet seat or a singing baked bean tin), it is not difficult to recognise a profound healing underneath the seemingly silly story.

It is the *objects* which seem to give the writing the power. I think that the imagined object speaks symbolically of the hidden treasure within; the subconscious speaks in symbol and metaphor, and objects are images. (Interestingly the object has been 'given' randomly by somebody else in the group.) As with all writing exercises, it is important that people don't feel judged or that they are competing with each other, so it needs handling sensitively, and as lightly as possible. It can sometimes be a relief to have some laughter and silliness after sessions which evoke tears, however healing and welcome those tears.

Objects from dreams or spiritual gifts given in visualisations can give particularly powerful messages from the deep subconscious. I have experienced this very powerfully for myself in a workshop led by Gillie Bolton.

Karen Hayes (1999, 2005) and Lesley Glaister (2004), respectively, introduced these next exercises to me. Both exercises make use of actual objects in order to enhance the development of plot and character in creative writing. In each case, before we began writing, we looked and handled actual objects and described them before trying the exercises. Karen asked us to imagine that this object was highly significant to our character. When were they given it? Or, our character finds this object. What memories does it evoke?

Lesley Glaister asked us to imagine why our character would steal this object.

These exercises work on the same principle: human beings give great metaphorical and totemic power to objects. For creative writing, it certainly helps make writing more concrete. In an odd way, in writing we are inverting the sculptor's process: a sculptor can turn intangible feelings into a three-dimensional object, whereas writing from an object helps to reconnect and communicate directly with intangible and complex feelings.

Two Creative Writing Activities: Using Plasticine and Personal Objects *Fiona Hamilton*

I used these two activities in creative writing workshops with different groups, one in a hospital, the other with a community group of elderly people with mental health needs. Both groups met over several weeks, and these activities took place a few sessions into each series. With the first group, the sense of touch provided a way into sensory and imaginative experience. With the second, personal objects enabled people to become tellers of their own stories.

Plasticine

I brought in some balls of different-coloured plasticine arranged on a dish. I put this in the centre of the room at the beginning of the session.

Each person was invited to take a ball of plasticine and mould it into something. I explained that they would be handing it on to someone else in the group when they had made it.

We sat modelling the plasticine for 15 minutes in silence. This gave enough time for people to get really involved with moulding and shaping the plasticine. People made: a basket, a shape that looked like a sun or a flower, a small curled-up shape, a piece curved into an arch, a cup and a horseshoe. Participants were then invited to pass their object to the person on their right, who was asked to notice how they felt receiving it, and then to do something to it – they could change it, add to it or remove from it. We placed the plasticine objects in the centre of the room.

After this, it was time for writing. Participants were given 15 minutes to write freely – I invited them to allow their thoughts to flow. We had a tea break, and then returned to share writing.

Writing included the following:

- The recipient of the basket imagined and made different things it could contain – eggs, fruit, flowers. She wrote about what it was like to receive a gift.

- The sun inspired the idea of it rotating in space like thoughts revolving in the writer's mind; its power and strength as a life-giving force, its worship by ancient civilisations, and also its capacity to overwhelm.

- The small curled-up shape was interpreted as a newborn baby, or even before birth. The writer wrote about feelings of protectiveness towards it, and her sense of its fragility.
- The arch shape was seen as a bridge, and the writer considered bridges between people and what happened when there was no bridge, how difficult it could be to build one, like trying to building it out of matchsticks and leaves.

Comments about the activity included:

> When she gave it to me, it seemed to be so right for me, it's just what I've been thinking about recently.

> It reminded me of being a child – I haven't touched plasticine for ages.

> I didn't know what the shape was at first, and then it looked like a baby.

> I didn't want to change it, it was so carefully made.

> I completely changed it.

> It's amazing how everyone makes something so unique.

> It was a bit like something growing and changing when I started to work on it.

A personally important object

I asked a group of elderly people to bring in an object that was important to them – something fairly small and portable. It could be an everyday object, something precious, a photo or something they carried around with them.

At the next session, most people had remembered to bring an object; two had not – I asked them if they had anything on them that they could use, or if not, could they remember an object and visualise it. The objects included: a plastic key-ring in the shape of a policeman, a china cup, a photo of grandchildren, a shell and a stone.

I then invited people to pass their object around the group and then, when it had come back to them, to tell us about it. The act of passing the object around contributed to group trust and involvement, as well as being affirming to the owner of it, who received interested, curious and appreciative comments about it.

I highlighted some of the information they might include when telling the group about their object, such as:

- its appearance, texture, and other features
- where and when they got it
- whether it was associated with any particular place or person
- whether they had ever lost it
- how they felt about it now.

People willingly spoke about their objects – they became spontaneous storytellers:

- The key-ring, carried around in the owner's handbag, made her feel protected.
- The china cup had been bought in a seaside town, where the owner had spent her honeymoon.
- The photo of grandchildren – the owner told the group the children's names, ages, what they liked doing, what they did when they came to visit.
- The stone was one of a collection the owner had made during travels around the world for his job as an engineer.

The next part of the activity was to write about the object. Here another dimension emerged, as people connected more with feelings and memories evoked by their objects, encouraged by the interest others had shown in their spoken stories.

- The key-ring owner 'talked to' her policeman, bringing out the humour in his cartoon appearance, and touching on her own feelings of vulnerability.
- The china cup became a meditation on memories of the writer's husband and grief that he was no longer alive. She described in detail the place where they had spent happy times.
- The stone allowed the writer to re-travel the world as he had done when younger, and to share some of his adventures with others.

Later, participants were able to photograph their objects with a digital camera and see the images on a laptop computer. For many of these elderly people it was the first time they had used such equipment and they found it exciting and affirming. Although with many groups the emphasis is on process rather than product, this group decided to produce a booklet of their images and poems. Many of them expressed pride in the finished work, and pleasure that they were able to take the booklet home and show it to others. I was moved and inspired by the wealth of life experience brought to these sessions and expressed in spoken and written words and pictures.

Empty Box   *Glynis Charlton*

I used this exercise when working with a group of six carers, ranging in age from their late forties to mid-seventies, five of whom were women. Some of the group were former carers, others were still caring for a relative at home. Most of them had briefly met one another before, at the monthly coffee mornings, but this was the first time they had come together in a creative writing class.

We met for a couple of hours on seven Thursday afternoons, in a comfortable meeting room, with refreshments freely on hand. One of the group (a lady in her early seventies) had an arts degree and had several small, published articles to her name. Another lady had some experience of writing for public speaking, whilst a third was still writing the occasional poem as a way of dealing with her bereavement. The remaining three members of the group had written nothing creative since school.

My series of workshops formed part of a residency with a literature resource centre and was arranged in partnership with Social Services. Although it wasn't essential, they had told me it would be good if I could draw out some of the issues around being a carer, the objective being to produce a small booklet for Carers Week. I knew that if I took a direct approach, most of the group would probably just walk out of the door. This had to be handled very sensitively.

I spent the first session or two using basic exercises around location and character, gradually getting them comfortable with the general idea of writing and sharing their work (although they were given the option of keeping their writing private if they wished). By the third session, certain issues had begun to emerge, such as feelings of loneliness and isolation, the longing for times past, the hope of better things to come or the guilty feelings associated with respite. Their writing had also begun to open up, develop and enter a different level. The lady who wrote poetry was producing some particularly evocative pieces. The one man in the group, who had tended to write about his past jobs, was now writing some poignant war memories and other pieces touching on his emotions, which he felt unable to share with the group but felt he wanted to show to me.

On week four I took along a tiny empty box, about four square centimetres. It was made of rough cream recycled material, with a small gold star on the lid, and was the smallest of a stack of three from my dressing table. I think I was probably influenced by the visualisation exercises at the back of Myra Schneider's *Writing My Way Through Cancer* (2003) plus my own imagination's tendency to 'shrink down' and explore tiny hidden worlds.

I placed the box out of reach in the middle of the workshop table. Some said how lovely it was, all were curious about its contents. While they were chatting, I put the kettle on. Then I began the exercise:

- Forget its size.[1] This box contains something very special to you. It can be real, imaginary, solid or abstract – anything you like – but the lid of the box is sealed and you can't get to it. What's in the box? What's it like not being able to get hold of it? Write about it in any way you wish for five or six minutes.

- Now you can suddenly get into the box and you take off the lid to touch what's inside. What's this like? (Another five minutes.)

- Take something from inside *you* that makes you feel angry or sad – a negative emotion – place it in the box, put the lid on and seal it down, out of sight, out of touch. If you wish, spend two or three minutes writing about how this feels.

I then took the box from the table and put it away in my bag. People sat back in their chairs with a sigh, smiled at one another and said, 'Phew…blimey' Clearly they had found it quite intense, but I had taken care to keep a watchful eye open for anyone becoming upset, and everyone had been writing constantly throughout. At this juncture, I said it was definitely time for a cup of tea and we chatted about the experience. Whilst one or two said it was tough, all agreed that it had been fascinating and

---

1   I cited a big jar of Marmite (yeast spread), since we'd just been sharing a joke about somebody's love of it, which would of course never fit inside the box.

most said they'd surprised themselves, writing about things they had never expected.

One person wrote about air and how, without it, there was no life – so the box wasn't empty, it was actually as full as it could possibly be. Another wrote about the memories of a loved one and how these could never actually be sealed away out of reach. Similarly, somebody else wrote about a very special photograph, another about her engagement ring. Not surprisingly, nobody wanted to share the negative emotion that they had sealed in the box.

After the tea break, I made sure I kept the rest of the session comparatively light hearted. They could each write a letter to a TV celebrity of their choice whom they particularly disliked.

At the following session, two people brought me poems they had felt compelled to write during the week, which they said were prompted by the box exercise. One was about society not knowing how to deal with bereaved people and another was about the theft of time.

Roman Story; Feather and Stone   *Geraldine Green*

As a tutor on a recent storytelling course run by an adult education Skills for Life Strategy, I worked with a group of women and one man, all of whom had little experience of writing and performing, apart from the man who wrote short stories.

There were two strands to the course: to encourage the group to think about what storytelling was and to work towards a Level 2 certificate in literacy. The course was spread over 15 weeks, two hours each week, and took place in a local library.

Most of the group were reluctant even to read aloud work written by other people, let alone to write and read their own; I felt a few gentle exercises were needed and I took along my djembe.

The drum acted like magic! The group began to open up; one, who had remained quiet during the first couple of sessions, suddenly blossomed and told the group how she had been on a course which used a drum and that she wrote poetry. The following week she read one of her poems out. I'd taken the drum in to explore rhythm in poetry and was amazed at how it acted as a liberator.

Making use of the space in the library helped. I made a point of using a more formal area of tables and chairs when we were writing or using the flip chart, moving to the brighter children's area tables when we were performing, sharing and reading.

The two most popular exercises were the Roman Story and Feather and Stone.

Roman Story

Two of the group worked in the local Roman museum and we visited it one week, took notes, looked at artefacts – such as togas, fish oil, jewellery, spears etc. – then the following week wrote pieces based on our visit. I asked the whole group to bring along togas and props for us to wear. I suggested something along the lines of an advert for a stonemason, a travel agent or the opening of an Italian restaurant. One of the group had the brilliant idea of an advert for a stonemason to build a long wall!

To get things going I wore a toga, gave a drum roll and did an 'Oyez! Oyez! New Ristorante opening in town!' I then asked the group to split into smaller groups, to write something, dress up and perform it.

They did this with enthusiasm! One group wrote an advert for a travel agent, one for an estate agent; each group dressed in togas, banged the drum and immersed themselves in playacting. It was great fun and the whole group, on their feedback forms, wrote how much they'd enjoyed it and how dressing up had helped them overcome feeling self-conscious. Although one, I think, felt a little silly in a toga, she still banged the drum and took part. It created a great atmosphere, very informal and great fun!

Each of them later remarked that it gave them confidence for the remainder of the course. I asked them to write a longer piece about their visit to the museum. One wrote a 'letter home' as a young soldier going into the army:

> Dear Remus
>
> … I'm trying not to worry too much about what lies ahead for me, but it's such unknown territory. I just don't know if I'll have the stamina to get through the training, never mind when I've got to go into battle… I don't think I can do this, I really don't. If I fail I will bring such shame on my family. I know you would be telling me to have faith in myself, but without you by my side, friend, I do worry about not coping. But I must stand by my decision…
>
> Your friend, Romulus

Feather and Stone

Whilst the Roman Story was an outward, active way of encouraging the group to write and read, the Feather and Stone exercise was a more inward form of guided imagery. I'm not sure where the idea came from, but I have all kinds of natural objects in my study that I use in writing exercises, to encourage people to use all their senses when writing, especially touch.

I asked each of them to bring in feathers and stones. I wanted the group to imagine themselves as the bird whose feather they had brought along, what it was like to be a bird or stone and to tell its story.

As in the Roman Story, I wanted to explore the idea of the 'other' – possibly another culture, country, language, religion, bird or inanimate object – and to heighten awareness and empathy towards the 'other'.

I asked the group to imagine a beautiful place: what they could see, smell, taste, touch and hear there. It was gentle, guided imagery allowing them to let go, allowing images and ideas to surface.

Each one of the group wrote some very moving pieces; sensitive and sometimes, I think, unexpected to themselves.

Fool's Gold *by Gloria Wood*

Sharp jagged edged
Gold glittery corners,
How beautiful am I
Shimmering beneath the morning sky.
Fool to pick me up
Fool to walk on by.
You may think I'm just fool's gold
But in me there's a story as yet untold.

Stone *by Anon*

I lie here now just filling a gap,
if only people knew how important I used to be.
I cry out to them as they pass,
but they never hear.
At most they stand on me
or soak me in water,

but never treat me with the respect I deserve,
I've even been picked up and thrown around.

Reflecting

I'd like to finish by reflecting on why both exercises appealed and stimulated the group, even though one was extrovert, group-centred and playful, the other more introspective and individual. My feeling is that the Roman Story enabled people to step behind the masks of history and personas, to help them empathise with people from another time and place and relate it to the present. The Feather and Stone exercise enabled people to make an inward journey, gently helping them take time out for themselves in a safe environment.

Finally...comments from the group:

> I want to help children and teenagers [to get] through bullying and to develop my own writing and poetry skills.

> I feel pleased with some of the work I've done; having read and performed to the group and written a few short stories I've shocked myself, not in the past realising I could do this.

Writing Self and Place   *Helen Boden*

The setting was unashamedly elegant: the anteroom to the Georgian ballroom at a book fair. This site-specific exercise is a practical demonstration of the relationships between creative writing and personal or therapeutic writing, between internal and external creative stimuli, and between individual and group. Previous groups in other places had found inspiration in flaking paint, filing cabinets and light switches. This space boasted pillars, chandeliers, ornate plasterwork, mirrors, a grand fireplace and a split-level parquet floor. Its size enabled different phases of the exercise to happen in different zones. Next door, other events at the fair included talks by James Kelman and George Galloway, and workshops on 'Creative Writing for Activists' and 'The Writing Cure v. the Talking Cure'.

About a dozen people turned up, not at all bad for a sunny Sunday morning in June. Most didn't yet know each other, or me. We introduced ourselves. There was a mix of experienced and confident writers, people both familiar and unfamiliar with holistic approaches to creativity, and interested but apprehensive beginners. As one part of the exercise involved some gentle movement, I checked if anyone had mobility problems.

We began, sitting in a semicircle, closing our eyes and turning our attention inwards. Focusing on our breath and heartbeat, the bodily rhythms that inspire the rhythms of our writing, we scanned our own bodies. When we opened our eyes, we wrote down a list of five adjectives that best described us, physically, mentally, emotionally or spiritually, in the present moment.

Next we moved away from our seats to stand in a circle, looking straight ahead, maintaining a loose, wide-angled view of what was in front, rather than focusing sharply on something specific. I invited everyone slowly to drop their heads until they were looking at the floor, and then rotate their heads and bodies, eyes still open, as far as they could without straining. At this point they began to raise their heads, and let their eyes travel up towards the ceiling, then across it, back down to the floor and finally up again to the centre. Then we repeated the movement in the opposite direction. We turned around to face outside the circle and performed the rotation again in both directions, noticing throughout whatever was passing before our eyes. Now everyone wrote, next to their adjective list, a list of five nouns, names of objects seen whilst glancing around the room. This was the trickiest bit for me. I told the 12 expectant faces, 'This stage of the exercise works best if you partially fold your paper over your adjective list, so this doesn't "influence" your writing of the noun list.' Fortunately I managed to demonstrate clearly so no one became anxious about getting the origami part of the exercise wrong!

The technique generated a list of five phrases, such as 'tired cornice' or 'excited radiator'. Now everyone read out their combinations, and I wrote these up on the whiteboard. Examples ranged from unintentionally literal or plausible ('broken arm', 'hungover curtain') to seemingly bizarre and unworkable ('elated doorknob', 'twisted clipboard'), and the pooling of phrases produced a lot of laughter. Everyone selected three phrases in preparation for the next stage: to incorporate each into a (separate) sentence. I asked, 'Under what circumstances or in what context might a clipboard be twisted?', and encouraged more confident writers to experiment grammatically by incorporating their phrase somewhere other than at the beginning of the sentence.

Then everyone read out their 'favourite' sentence, which was written up. We discussed which sentences from the collection might make a good story opening and conclusion. We spent some time thinking about how to go about making the choice, checking that everyone was comfortable with their own level of participation. It was delightful to witness people instinctively 'caring' for each other and encouraging less confident writers. I often think that creative writing involves a combination of making conscious choices and allowing chance to intervene. Here we found our opening sentence, 'The *tired mirror* reflected the many faces', by drawing straws. The closing sentence was voted on, and the winner was 'In the *detached light* of morning, she finally understood.'

Everyone now retreated into their own space to write a story that connected up the agreed beginning and ending. As our anteroom also doubled as the book fair café, everyone had the luxury of their own table. I suggested they write the opening sentence at the top of an A4 sheet and the closing one at the bottom, and allowed about 30 minutes before everyone reconvened in the circle, to reflect upon the experience, and read their stories and receive feedback if they wished. As the café was now opening for lunch, we had an audience – not usually something to be recommmended, but as everyone had been warned about this in advance, and written fictions considerably removed from the personal starting points, confidentiality and privacy weren't a problem. Everyone read, and received enthusiastic applause.

I initially developed Writing Self and Place for a 'Writing for Well-being' course which I have run in a number of settings, including an educational/leisure project for carers and a community centre. I also use it, in abbreviated form, as a day workshop warm-up. Its 'adjective + noun' formula for generating writing seems quite common: I've encountered a number of variants. I was interested in ways of developing the word game by grounding it in personal embodied experience, and extending it, via a collective collaborative practice, through a series of incremental stages, into the production of an original creative piece. On this occasion selves intermeshed with place to inspire some of the most engaging work I have heard produced in a two-hour workshop.

Mirror, Mirror by Chris Korycinski

The tired mirror reflected the many faces and conversations held within her frame. The gold was tarnished, the silvering speckled and pitted. Brightness, darkness; reflection, hollowness. The history of the family was embodied in her being, and she had served the family well, showing them the faces of hope and happiness even whilst the reality of life gnawed away at them. But a good servant will make sacrifices and be repaid with the knowledge that work has been done well and faithfully, that fears and terrors which oppressed her owners were able to flow away through the images of light and joy reflected back.

But last night was different.

She could see from her commanding position in the hallway that furniture was being moved out, that the house – after over 400 years – was being closed down. The mournful echoes of people's voices told her that most of the house was now empty, barren, merely a shell. The owners had left and there was no one to stand in front of her and gaze at themselves; she could no longer perform any service for them.

She looked down and saw men coming nearer and nearer towards her – where could they take her? Where would she go? Whom should she serve? Then she saw that each man carried an axe, and in the detached light of the early morning, she finally understood.

The Loss *by Marloes van Ameron*

The tired mirror reflected the many faces
And conversations held within its frame.
Her first inclination was to smash it, destroy all those
painfully precious memories,
Scatter and send the mirror to the floor
Into 100,000 pieces
And stamp them to death, each individually.
Now that he was gone, what good would a reminder do?
It seemed to her that life had become cohesionless, without
any sense of meaning anymore.
Why continue to go through the motions one-by-one
When in the end all that counts is the baggage of love we
carry around with us
But then have to give up as we depart?

Looking in the mirror again, she could just see his loving face
and the many
Connecting conversations they had had spring back to life:
The flood of joy they had bathed in during his stay,

That rush of love, hope and passion that kept on connecting
them over time –

This heritage of memories needed to be nurtured as a precious
treasure.

In the detached light of morning she finally understood.

Feeling, Smelling, Hearing, Tasting Perhaps, But Not Seeing
Gillie Bolton
with Catherine Byron and Robert Hamberger

One of my very first introductions to writing workshops was with poet
Catherine Byron. It was many years ago, but such a vital memory it is still
vivid in my mind.

There were only about eight of us sitting in a circle. We were all writers
(in my case would-be writer) on a writers' training course of some sort
funded by the Arts Council. The co-facilitator was there too, but he is
shadowy in my memory: it was Catherine who held the power.

She explained that she was going to give us an object to feel, smell,
make sounds from, taste if we wished, but not see. She promised not to give
us anything in the least nasty.

We sat with our hands together in our laps, eyes closed waiting like
supplicants. She came gently round the room placing an object in each pair
of hands. Mine was large, heavy and cold, egg-shaped but with an uneven
surface. The process excited me, while making me slightly anxious.

While I held my object, I could hear people pinging and scratching:
they clearly had very different things to mine. After about five minutes with
our objects, Catherine collected the pieces from opened palms, going the
same way round the room to give us each an equal amount of time with our
thing. It was only when she had stowed them all back in her bag that she
told us to open our eyes. Whether anyone peeped I don't know. I got to
know Catherine after that, and she showed me my beachcombed fishing-
net weight; I wouldn't have seen it otherwise.

Still without speaking we were asked to take up pen and paper and
write whatever came into our heads from the experience. This is what
I wrote:

Love Charm by *Gillie Bolton*

My hands were cupped
open to receive the gift you gave me
with no knowledge of its weight,
heavy on my upturned palms
old and deep and cold
but not so cold as when you took it
from the earth
warmed it with your body,
this near-sphere
is pierced through its roughness
for me to wear

I carry its weight lightly.

(Looking back from nearly 20 years later, I think the gift Catherine gave me
was the gift of poetry.)

Then we read our writing to each other and commented supportively,
and made suggestions for rewriting. Catherine said she thought my poem
was a *gift*, and did not need rewriting.

I have used this workshop idea many times since, having beachcombed
my own objects, scrubbing and boiling them so I know they are quite clean.
Though Catherine is astonished I do this and says, 'I am very keen on the
sense of smell, and have always made sure my sea-bag is salty and sandy
and refreshed every so often with new smelly seaweed, and that my
attic/skip-bag is always dusty and grotty!'

As well as writing about the object, I have found that many people have
written about the experience of waiting to be given something; they've
expressed anxiety and jealousy that others had received before them and
that some might have nicer things than they did. All these feelings are those
of children being given food or gifts: good to remember and work on, and
then to move on from again. Some people have compared it to communion:
waiting for the wafer of life.

Catherine made the whole process comfortable yet dynamic. I can't
remember any difficulty on that occasion with anyone being nervous of
closing their eyes. She says now:

> The requirement that eyes be closed can cause anxieties,
> especially for some contact lens wearers. If someone is clearly in

difficulties about it, I ask them to handle their object behind their back, and – of course – to try not to see others' objects. Over the years many anxious people have dropped their objections when I've offered them the behind-back option, and almost all of these have in fact closed their eyes and received it like the rest. And sometimes those who have taken it behind their back find that they want so much to smell and taste their object that they close their eyes and bring it round to the front!

When I have done this workshop I introduce the closing of the eyes carefully, giving people clear permission to keep their eyes open if they feel uncomfortable with it. Like Catherine I have found that offering an opt-out from the beginning does seem to reduce anxiety; I don't think anyone has ever refused to close their eyes. I also ask them to open their eyes at the end slowly, bringing them back into the world of light and normal companionship carefully.

Recently Robert Hamberger, a friend and poet colleague of both Catherine and myself, led a writing exercise for our poetry group. It was the same kind of process with the difference that there were very few of us, and we know each other very well. He gave me a fake pearl necklace of his mother's. I wrote about how I'd just had my pearls restrung for my daughter, around whose delicate throat they look utterly beautiful. I never wore them as they symbolised 'twin-set and pearls' – the dreadful image of the *young lady* I was brought up to be. It was an extremely angry and useful piece of writing.

A Gift of Pearls by Gillie Bolton

They weren't mine
though my seven-year self received them
in a box inlaid with my initials,
a certificate recording every pearl,
and an unspoken message:

When you grow up you will wear these
dusted with face powder, doused with Chanel
over a muted shade of cashmere,
your manicured nails will constantly check
the largest lies in the hollow of your throat.

These pearls were the gift of oysters
capturing the sea's light,
now I give them to my daughter
who wears them with jeans, wonky
around her naked throat.

Robert watched me sightlessly and frustratedly trying to close the necklace clasp, and wrote a powerful sonnet about hooking his mother's frock up for her to go out on a Friday night, and the odd role mix this was. His mother was a single parent and he was being the man of the house. As facilitator, watching people sensing their objects, I too have written about the experience alongside my group, and found it very rewarding.

Hook and Eye by *Robert Hamberger*

'Can you do me up?' She turns her back,
her shoulders bare, dress with its zip
an inch undone, the hook and eye a gap,
needing me to strain that silver link,
to latch its tiny horseshoe, lock
together. Can I close this clasp to help
those glad-rags hold her in? The air's sharp
with hairspray, scent dabbed at her neck
and wrists. It's a fiddly race
to clinch it before she'll snap and moan.
I'm fingers and thumbs. If I fix it her voice
stays happy, ready to paint the town,
this bolder version of my mother, her face
turning to me, smiling, thanking her son.

Robert has added this:

I somehow 'knew' instinctively that the pearls would be the right object to give you. Knowing you made this easier, but I've also found that the workshop leader can usefully follow their instinct about which object to give to unknown writers. An example I remember is that I gave one writer a feather. It turned out that she had distressing memories as a child of feeding her grandmother's chickens, so holding the feather was initially very difficult for her. However, it led to a powerful poem that began: 'Black cold fear – Granny's farm, Red, Brown chickens clucking chasing'. Unknown to the workshop leader, an object may spark associations for a writer that are distressing and the workshop leader must be ready to support the writer with making a shape and sense of that distress, if possible.

Pictures, Coloured Paper and Pens, Buttons and Skulls
Gillie Bolton

Pictures are a stimulus used by most facilitators I would guess. Ways to use them are as varied as the people. My huge collection is from calendars, birthday and Christmas cards, postcards from exhibitions and sent by friends. When I need them I riffle through for inspiration – conversation pieces for example. Recently I very successfully sorted out a pile which seemed all to be about weather. I used them as an ice-breaker with a new group which was to last three days. We all selected an image, or rather allowed an image to choose us. We then each chose a weather picture for every other member of the group (if it's a large group you can split them into small groups for this), and presented it to them. Participants were encouraged not to articulate reasons for their choice, still less to tell the other person if they did have an idea why they'd chosen a particular image. We then wrote about whichever picture we wanted to, and the whole experience. (For another, more intensive exercise, see Bolton and Stoner 2004.)

Coloured paper and pens have often given me a gentle opener for the first flow writing, particularly for the doctors and nurses I generally work with; it goes a little way to breaking the tension of 'Oh dear I can't write!' Participants are usually very definite about which colour they want, sometimes squabbling over the last purple or yellow sheet.

Yellow is supposed to be the creative colour. Several doctors who have become committed writers since my workshops habitually use yellow pads. They feel it helps. The colours of the photocopy paper I use tend to be a bit *loo-paper* though some darker colours are available – aquamarine and purple for example. Coloured paper and pens can create a simple warm-up exercise for either adults or children: 'Write a blue, purple or yellow thought.'

I have run many workshops with buttons (Bolton 1999), shells (Bolton 2000), hats (see Bolton 1999, 2005) and varied containers (Bolton 2001).

I don't think I've written about using skulls, of which I have a large collection (sheep, mouse, blackbird, snake, stag…), but the time I remember best was with a young man with a diagnosis of schizophrenia. His writing, imaginatively crawling into the sheep's skull, was an exploration into the inside of his own skull; it was quite remarkable and very useful to him.

A warm-up ice-breaker exercise I've happily used was with imaginary objects. Everyone sits in a circle; I start by cupping my hands as if holding something precious, and carefully hand this imaginary object to the person beside me. They receive it, turn it into something else and hand it to the person next to them, and so on round the circle until it reaches me again. It has to be done very fast in order not to become boring, and is touching and hilarious in turns.

CHAPTER 4

Writing from Published Poems

Edited by Victoria Field

There is a long tradition of using published poems as a springboard for therapeutic writing. The 'biblio-poetry therapy' model established in the United States dates from the 1930s and typically has three stages (Mazza 1993). First, the therapist or facilitator will introduce a text of some kind to the group or client and invite reflection on its contents. Often, the simpler the text, the more complex the responses. The text is usually a poem but can be any other short, intense piece of writing, or even a recording of a song or a film clip, that has the potential of eliciting an emotional response. There are many favourite poems for using in this context and one of their characteristics is that they can be interpreted or re-interpreted time and again from many different perspectives.

Then, a writing activity or exercise based on the text will be suggested. Again, depending on the group, this may be more or less complex. The third stage is the sharing of the pieces of writing and discussion and reflection on them in their own right. The sharing of the writing done in response to the presented poem is often where the most insight occurs.

The field of poetry therapy is a large and growing one with many related practices, such as journalling or diary writing. Here, we provide some workshop examples that use poetry therapy techniques but recommend that if you are interested in this area you should contact the National Association for Poetry Therapy for further details and a reading list (see Appendix 3 for contact information).

In this chapter, Roselle Angwin describes using a classic poem, Wallace Stevens' 'Thirteen Ways of Looking at a Blackbird', with her advanced poetry group and with teenage boys, showing how a powerful poem can work with very distinct groups. Although she is not working explicitly therapeutically, the poem encourages a sense of contemplation of our role in the natural and spiritual world. She also describes her anxiety at using a 'difficult' poem. The choice of poem to bring to a group is of crucial importance and requires careful thought and preparation. Sometimes, though, hostility to a poem in a group setting can be a useful response as it can highlight aspects of more general emotional responses. How to work with such different reactions is part of the poetry therapist's training. Miriam Halahmy's writing group also worked with the same Wallace Stevens poem. Miriam takes it further by using the poetic responses as a stimulus to yet more writing which focused on more personal issues. This can be useful for building a sense of cohesion in the group but is a technique to be used with care as sometimes people feel uncomfortable at their work being appropriated. Again, in Miriam's example, the writers gained unexpected personal insight through their writing.

Sherry Reiter's workshop description focuses on a well-known Rumi poem. This is a good example of a poem that, through the metaphor of a person as 'guest house' for emotions, can be a springboard for many kinds of discussion or writing. In this instance, Sherry focuses on depression and the examples she gives of participants' writing show clearly how individuals can respond to a poem and make it their own, some choosing to write more generally and abstractly, others using concrete imagery. Patricia L. Grant uses the same poem as a stimulus both to introduce the idea of poetry therapy but also to create a group poem. Asking people to contribute lines or images whilst the facilitator scribes is a way of introducing writing or poetry to people who may have difficulty with the physical act of writing itself. I have used this technique with many groups in different settings, including infants, the elderly and learning disabled adults. There is often a great sense of pride in a group poem which can be greater than the sum of its parts.

Fiona Hamilton describes a session with cancer patients in which she invites them to write from a line of a poem they have shared. This simple suggestion is immensely effective in allowing people to write 'what they need to write'. Fiona's piece also exemplifies the necessary facilitator skills of allowing participants to disclose as much or as little as they wish and creating an atmosphere for the safe expression and release of complex emotions. One way in which poetry facilitates understanding of self and others is through the use of metaphor. The workshop described by Elaine Trevitt shows how metaphor can be playful and at the same time reveal deeper truths. By turning abstract emotions into creatures, the writers in this workshop are able to stand back and reflect on the roles important emotional states play in their lives.

Dominic McLoughlin works in health- and social-care settings but concentrates on how the process of studying poetry writing can be of value for its own sake and encourage new ways of framing the world.

Our final piece, contributed by Leone Ridsdale, is a description of a workshop given by John Fox, in which she reflects on the experience from the point of view of a participant. Everyone in the workshop would have described the experience differently and this subjective view is immensely valuable – facilitators can gain important insights when they read such accounts.

The Dot of the I   *Roselle Angwin*

The opening stanza of Wallace Stevens' powerful poem 'Thirteen Ways of Looking at a Blackbird' (Stevens 1982, p.421) immediately creates a vivid picture describing how against an immense, snowy landscape of twenty mountains, with their implicit silence and stillness, the single moving thing was the blackbird's eye. Not the expected blackbird, note, but just the eye of the blackbird; a detail that enhances the sense of snowy vastness. This moving thing is something so minute as surely to be totally invisible; and yet, the poem implies, that tiny dot is also all-seeing.

That huge whiteness and the dot of blackness also conjure an atmosphere of juxtaposition, and set up some kind of creative tension for us. Maybe an emotional response also happens: a sense of immense stillness and waiting (exploded with the sudden whirling movement in stanza II); maybe our response is one of loneliness, or dread; maybe one of anticipation.

The opening of stanza II, where an 'I' is introduced, suggests a further realisation of the metaphor: our tiny human life against that vastness. So we are invited to question: which eye is he talking about? The eye/I of the blackbird, or the new 'I'? Who is doing the looking?

I have loved that poem for over 20 years. Another thing I love, both as a writer and as a course facilitator, is that moment when connections are made. I don't just mean an understanding; but a realisation of the points at which inner and outer worlds come together. What happens when the blackbird and the observer of the blackbird and the landscape all fuse in the imagination; where 'eye' and 'I' meet; and then meet with the man, woman and blackbird whom Stevens tells us 'are one' in stanza IV? What happens when we as reader or listener participate as another 'I/eye'?

Much of my work is directed towards finding ways to enable this sense of connection and, as a creative writing facilitator with a strong belief in the power of the word to transform people, I am also always looking for new ways into the creative process; ways that will change, however minutely, the perception of the participants.

A few months ago I led a workshop with my regular advanced poetry group ('Two Rivers') using that poem as a model. Although it is not overtly a 'writing for personal development' group, every member is aware that there is a crossover. When you work for many years with the same group of people in the context of poetry, something alchemical happens, and what is shared in the group is often deeply intimate stuff for which there may be no other room anywhere in the busy outer world.

We read the poem in turns, several times. Then we talked about it at length, for maybe two hours (could have been all day). Afterwards, I suggested that they found a way to write, using that poem as a model, from their own experience. I set them four tasks:

- to keep each stanza very short and the language strong but simple
- to write anything between 5 and 15 stanzas
- to ensure that the subject of the poem appeared in some way in each stanza
- to include themselves in the poem.

I suggested that it was a matter for personal choice whether they followed Stevens' sequence or departed from it.

Below is an extract from one of the pieces from the twelve or so members of that group. Ostensibly about a particular woman, it is actually about the soul, or in this case the anima of the poet concerned (he told us).

13 Ways of Looking at Her by *Brian King*

I ran along her snow dunes
my hot blood blindfolded
she asked for my eyes

I was in three minds:
fox, express train, juggler
she worried about the desperate boy

she said she was a good catch
car, house, job, pension
I forgot my fishing rod

infinity was one area
she wouldn't inhabit
unless it was her infinity...

her instinct for self-preservation
gave her greater powers of deception
than I could ever have

it was a cold night
we huddled together in a damp cave
waiting for her to have the last word

A few weeks ago I opened a wonderful book by Christian McEwen and Mark Statman in the Teachers and Writers Collaborative series: *The Alphabet of the Trees* (2000). Having read a classroom piece on just that poem, I thought I would use it as a model for one of the classes when I was asked to return to the boys' school where I'd been poet-in-residence the previous winter. The lessons are only 35 minutes long, and I had two sessions: one for exploring the poem, one for their writing. At the time, that seemed fine – though I knew we really needed a lot longer.

On the morning, though, I woke up terrified. These were third formers – 13- and 14-year-olds! How dare I attempt to explore in half an hour the profundity of this poem with 24 young teenagers! It's a difficult enough poem for adults. Plus their class teacher, himself a poet, is a well-known figure in literary circles – and I am not a trained teacher. What could I have been thinking of? I arrived at the classroom door shaking.

I needn't have worried. After we had read it three times, the boys knew immediately and exactly what the poem was about. The connection had been made.

'It's about the imagination and how we fear it.'

'No, it's about the fact that fear stops our imagination, and that if we aren't afraid we can allow our imagination to fly like the blackbird, or flow like the river' [later in the poem].

'It's about how small we are and how big the universe is.'

'It's about the fact that we aren't any different from the blackbird, or from nature.'

'I think it's about the fact that in a world that's full of powerful white people we need to remember to see the black people too and not fear them.' [This, poignantly, from the only Asian in the classroom.]

And finally, and with the class's agreement: 'It's a poem about the soul.'

What's more, in lesson 2, every boy in that classroom wrote a poem; not only that, each wrote a good poem, a profound and unique poem exploring their place as the seeing 'I' in this unthinkably huge universe of ours.

Ways of Looking, Ways of Seeing   *Miriam Halahmy*

My Monday morning workshop happens to be all women; it just worked out that way and so we have created a women's group without even trying. The group has met weekly for a year and their writing experiences range from beginners to published writers.

As with Roselle's experience described above, the workshops described here grew out of Wallace Stevens' great poem, 'Thirteen Ways of Looking at a Blackbird'. I have always loved the poem. The single image of the blackbird which threads throughout the poem is a powerful tool in my exploration of the role of the subconscious in creative writing. Five members of the group went through the whole process.

In the first session we read the text and discussed themes to trigger some writing. We decided to write poems on six or seven ways of looking at the wind, water, a painting, an apple tree, summer or a photograph. The group wrote in class and read back their first efforts. After some initial feedback, they continued with their work at home.

In the second session, when Anna read out the redraft of her poem, I suggested that she might like to change the order of her stanzas. 'Try cutting the poem up and rearranging the stanzas until you like the order.' Anna loved the idea. It was then that I suggested we take the idea further. Each participant would bring a typed version of their poems the following week. We would cut up the poems, put them in three piles with the stanzas of Stevens' poem, and then each choose three stanzas at random as a trigger for a piece of writing. The group thought this was an exciting idea.

Exploration of a theme from different angles, looking and reflecting on a deeper subconscious level, as opposed to working in a simpler, descriptive framework, encouraged the writers to take their writing forward in new directions. The exercise also freed them up to experiment with style and form.

The following week, armed with scissors, the group sliced through their poems, spread them across three piles and chose three stanzas each at random to work on. Some remarkable work emerged.

During this session Alison felt that the whole process had really stretched her imagination. She usually wrote factual pieces and this exercise stimulated her to write in a completely new direction. Here is the first stanza of the poem she wrote, based on a holiday in Portugal:

> Children laughing as the car swerves
> We cling to car and little ones
> As rain beats down lashing nerves
> Looking down the hill to the valley
> We hear the gulls cawing, crossing
> To and fro as lightning echoes across the mountains

Sue's poem on the wind moved from storms to kite flying and finished with:

> The flag is limp, it doesn't move, it has no inner strength
> it's crying out to be noticed it's really quite fed up
> suddenly its friend the wind gives it a small momentum
> it's waving now, really happy and Greece has won the cup

It was this quite cheerful stanza which Anna picked up. But Anna felt 'dried out' this week. The process had triggered memories of a time in her past when she felt 'like a limp flag'. She felt empty and alone:

> with no movement. I want to be seen and nurtured. Appreciated for who I am. What does not show like the black egg which precedes the golden one? I need to move, but fear sweeps my soul. I open the window and look out. A strong wind sweeps my face.

Sue's stanza had acted as a trigger to feelings and memories buried deep in Anna's subconscious and her piece of writing reflected the struggle with the 'black egg' and a strong determination to return to a more positive mood.

Another interesting development occurred in Janette's writing, which took her off at a new tangent, 'like a creature I had made'. Janette was normally an entertaining short story writer; this piece was like a roller coaster ride, written in short poetic lines. Janette herself was fascinated how this exercise had opened up a whole new aspect of her writing:

I went out
on the street I saw a drunk
lurching, shouting obscenities
I went back
got into my car
joined the thrusting, weaving
tearing mass along the motorway…

Leah, a teacher of dance and movement, had begun by writing about a river. She explained how dancing is her life. But she is always in two or three minds about what she wants to do, constantly asking herself, 'What is my future? Dancing, writing, painting?' She feels that her life is always weaving like a snake. During the time we spent on this theme, Leah wrote several poems, both in the workshops and at home, all of which explored these questions which she feels are central to her life today. An example is given below.

The gracious grey-silver snake
Winding in the valley

The river reflects the winding shapes
Of my spine

Trees grow in the river banks
Like dots in a landscape.

This is a multi-sensory approach to creative writing involving scissors, paper and glue; cutting, gathering and rearranging. The very physicality of this work created a strong and enabling atmosphere in the group, moving from the buzz of laughter and chat as they passed tools and materials, to a deep reflective silence when writing. Combining physical, creative and mental activities provided new opportunities to mine the rich vein of the subconscious.

The writers were both challenged by the process and led into hitherto unexplored territories of their lives by the writing experience which unfolded. Within such a process creative writing can provide a route forward for participants exploring the map of their inner worlds and experiences.

In the Guest House of the Heart *Sherry Reiter*

I would like to share an exercise that I used for the training of poetry therapists at The Creative Righting Center in New York City. The 12 trainees are all persons from various helping professions (creative arts therapists, social workers, counsellors, chaplains, educators and librarians). They are committed to attend a four-hour training one Sunday a month for the next two years. One hour is devoted to supervision. I facilitate a two-hour session and in the fourth hour one of the trainees facilitates a group. The trainees are participating in an experiential peer group, in which they are asked to fully immerse themselves in the creative process.

Today is the first session of the year. The focus is on the topic of depression. I begin the workshop with a brief role-play. Someone knocks on the door of the room. One of the trainees drapes a black sweater over her head and menacingly enters our space. 'What do you want?' I ask. She replies, 'I just want to be with you.' I ask the group, 'Who is this guest that just dropped in?' Without hesitation they identify it as Depression. Each person is asked for a one-word association to the word 'depression'. Then we read 'The Guest House' by Rumi (1995, p.109).

Participants are first given the directive to draw 'the guest house of their heart'. They are asked to delineate the rooms of their heart and the guests (emotions) that live there. Specifically, they are asked to describe the kind of room in which Depression lives. (Large? Small? Narrow?) Where does Depression reside? (In the attic, the basement or the living room?) After completing their drawings, they are asked to write about Depression and how it takes up its residency in their lives. Is depression a temporary vagrant, or has it taken up permanent residency? What kind of furniture is in this room? What sights, sounds, smells?

The writings which resulted were extraordinary in their vividness and were accompanied by brilliant drawings. Here are excerpts from three of them:

The Guest House by *Susan Wirth Fusco*

A visitor,
A sinewy line,
enters
through the front door,
unafraid,
like any other guest.

A black line of depression –
Hopelessness, Sorrow, Grief,
Helplessness –
enters any or every room.

Felicitous guest,
unwelcome stranger,
Depression wanders along and through
unknowing corridors, familiar hallways, and unsuspecting paths,
into spaces and places where it is not invited, not expected.

...I have learned that depression walks everywhere,
enters all rooms.
Courteously knocking? No, there is a
transcendentally
passing through – through iron doors, wooden doors,
locked doors, gated passageways...

Sit With Me by *Roselle P. O'Brien*

Depression sits with me in her chair.
I've had the chair since I was eight.
It's in storage now, the chair.
In a week I'll take it out and brush away the dust.

Depression rocked in the white chair with golden
leaves painted on the head rest.
It's a rocking chair,
Bigger than my sister's.

Better.
Its spot is in front of the closet door,
cosy on the midnight blue shag rug.

… Depression showed me
A place to get to if you rock just the right way,
or fast enough…
I never got it figured out.
Depression changed the rules and then stopped caring…

Depression would sit with me there
and we'd stare and stare into the three-way mirror
until my face became a monster's face,
then indistinct,
then black.
I miss the blue rug.

Where Is the Guest? by Kathryn M. Fazio

Depression resides in my bed.
It's a bed in my living room.
A cramped studio with a window of joy,
A tree I did not put there…

What a sanctuary of sorrow I lie on each night!
Mattress ruffles…invisible.
Only when I look out the window do I find joy.
Gratitude resurrected in a sanctuary constructed

Well before the menial concept of me.
I watch as empathy glows around a window,
Much greater than myself
Or the apathy I concern myself with.

And how is it, I would never treat any other person
With such a punitive ruler or measuring stick?
Pry them open.
Probe for value.

I love the rainbow
Above a bed I must leave.
It is true, I can no longer pay the rent on this dwelling.
And should I shoulder it to my next residence…

I pray gratitude will show up like a ditto mark and scatter
Into the room of chaos I call depression…

In the discussion following, we discussed the qualities of depression, which are multifaceted. Susan refers to the uninvited guest who passes through iron doors, wooden doors, locked doors, gated passageways. In Roselle's poem, Depression rocks in the rocking chair, comforting and comfortable because it is so familiar. Depression distorts one's own image: 'Depression would sit with me there/and we'd stare and stare into the three-way mirror/until my face became a monster's face.' In Kathryn's work, depression is a 'sanctuary of sorrow', a punitive place. 'And how is it, I would never treat any other person/With such a punitive ruler or measuring stick?' The issue of responsibility is raised.

Because this is a first meeting at the Creative Righting Center, we tread lightly because we do not know each other well. Feedback is given in broad strokes. I focus on the symbols of hope: the windows, gateways, empathy, the rainbow, gratitude. We are starting to listen for the messages in each person's personal code of imagery. Each member of the group shares their work. We are moved by each other's honesty and authenticity.

And how would Rumi feel about the way we've used his poem? I think he would be pleased to have served as 'our guide from beyond'!

How the 'Hang-Out Poets' Came to Be   *Patricia L. Grant*

I worked with those who had closed-head (i.e. non-penetrative) injuries. The severity of those kinds of injuries usually leave the patient in a coma, often lasting two or three months. Extensive rehabilitation is needed to retrain brain functions, so that the individual can relearn walking, speaking, using fine motor skills and redeveloping thinking skills. Frequently, these patients are unable to go back to work or to function effectively socially.

As a poetry therapist in training, I was finally given permission to try my wings and facilitate my own group. I contacted Craig Hospital which is renowned for its rehabilitation of closed-head injuries and spinal cord injuries. At first, the social workers involved in follow-up services said that what I proposed was not workable for their populations. However, Jan Nice, who runs the Hang-Out Group – an out-patient facility for people with closed-head injuries – said that poetry therapy might be workable for her patients.

But before I could be officially accepted by the Hang-Out Group, the board of directors, many of whom were closed-head injured, asked me to do a presentation for their entire group. There were 60 people present.

My own goals were to illustrate how poetry enhances lives, to demonstrate that writing poetry allows participants to develop an understanding of themselves and others, and to inspire participants so that they experienced the joy of creating their own poetry.

My first meeting with the Hang-Out Group lasted two hours. My warm-up exercise was to have everyone close their eyes and picture a guest house or a guest room. When they were ready, I asked questions of the group such as 'Where is your guest house/room?', 'What does your guest house/room look like?', 'Who stayed in your guest house/room?' and so on. All of the participants readily volunteered their answers. I then asked each of them to picture their own bodies as guest houses. I offered ideas, such as their guest houses could contain anger, love, generosity, people or events. Then I asked them to think about what each of them contained within their own body/guest house.

I followed these warm-ups by reading 'The Guest House' by Rumi (1995, p.109). All participants had their own copies of the poem to read from, as I read the poem to them. One of the participants volunteered to reread the poem. I then asked all the participants to volunteer ideas for what they would include in their guest houses. The replies came fast and furious. Hands went up everywhere. My assistant, Donna, wrote each response offered on a large flip chart. Each response was numbered. Donna could barely keep up. Each person had not just one word, but entire sentences to add to their guest house. One person even quoted from the poem itself, saying:

> When I woke up from my coma, 'my house was swept clean / empty of its furniture' and I was happy. God had protected me and will always protect me and every day offers me new delights.

Because we were running short of time, we were unable to call on all of those who wanted to speak. However, we did call on most of the participants. When finished with this part of the writing exercise, we filled five large flip-chart sheets with their responses. During the week, I put these responses together and typed them, so that the end result was a group poem. Later, eight members of this large group signed up for extended poetry therapy sessions.

The Guest House by the Hang-Out Group (31 March 2004)

In my guest house, I will invite love and God.
I will make room for grace and forgiveness.
I will have understanding.
I will make room for lifelong learning.
I will invite caring and compassion.

In my guest house, I will clean it of
unhappiness and negative emotions.
No one will judge others, and there will be no evil or hatred.
I will invite patience with all I meet.
I will be grateful for all those in my life who care about me.
I will have wellness and recuperation.
I will welcome studying and developing moral intellect...

In my guest house, I will have room
for three ample meals a day.
I will take time to give thanks for everything.
I will develop inner beauty.
I will have room for more friendships.
I will always have room for more love...

A Poem as a Beginning   *Fiona Hamilton*

The ingredients for this workshop came from different sources. Without knowing it, I had been harvesting them for a few weeks, so that when I came to prepare the session they came together readily.

I was to be working with a group of people with cancer, or affected by it, in an art room just big enough for a circle of 11 chairs, at a complementary health centre. This was to be the first of a series of four two-hour sessions, free to participants, funded by Writing in Healthcare, an organisation supported by Arts Council England and Awards for All.

The ingredients included my previous experiences of using 'Wild Geese' by Mary Oliver and 'The Lake Isle of Innisfree' by W.B. Yeats as starting points in previous workshops; poetry collections I was reading at the time – in particular the anthology *Staying Alive* published by Bloodaxe; the season – it was autumn; my own current writing interests; and my awareness of themes that resonate particularly with people with cancer, such as uncertainty, joy experienced in the moment, mortality, sadness, anger, hope and journeys.

I wanted to create a calm, holding, spacious and creatively interesting atmosphere for the group. I came across the poem 'The Language Issue' by Nuala ni Dhomhnaill in the anthology *Staying Alive* (2002, p.322), and felt that it could be a good starting point. The poem has a beauty and containment, as well as space for participants to interpret and respond in their own ways. Its abundance of nouns – boat, infant, basket, bitumen, river etc. – would provide variety and 'grounding' when it came to selecting words for their own writing. The theme of hope would be pertinent to this group and would allow room for more personal expression if participants wanted.

Also, the poem's themes would support something I wanted to say at the beginning of the workshop – that it takes courage to share one's writing with strangers, and that what we were about to do with words was experiment, not knowing where they would take us.

I arrived with my usual bag of equipment – clipboards, pens, paper. The chairs were arranged already, and there was a jug of cold water, plastic cups and tissues on the table by the door. I was welcomed by a member of staff and given a list of participants' names and name labels. These indications of practical and personal support contributed to my positive feelings as we assembled in the room.

After introducing myself to the group and mentioning some practical matters, I invited people to introduce themselves. Most had not attended a creative writing workshop before. Some had written diaries and poems. One had enrolled on a distance-learning writing course. One wrote song lyrics. One had written 'lots of reports but nothing creative'. Two said that they had started to want to write during cancer treatment.

I handed out the poem. We read it out, a line each around the circle, slowly. I then invited everyone to choose a phrase from the poem and use it as a first line for a piece of their own writing. I encouraged them not to aim for a 'finished product', just allow thoughts and feelings to flow. I gave 15 minutes of silence to write in.

At the end of 15 minutes, everyone had written something. There was the option not to read out, but everyone chose to.

The first participant had chosen the line referring to uncertainty about where the boat 'might end up'. This participant had written about 'not knowing' – about whether stepping into 'un-knowing' meant losing your power. Her piece ended with the phrase 'now that I know, what difference does it make?'.

I commented that the piece spoke about uncertainty and it asked a series of questions which appeared to be challenging commonly held assumptions. Someone else noted a tone of anger at the end of the piece. People discussed different aspects of having incomplete knowledge, and this feature of human existence being more obvious when one has cancer.

I felt that the first exchanges were affirming to the participant who had read out and were helping the group to gel. When someone asked the writer for more information about the 'facts' behind the piece, I intervened, asking if she wanted to provide them. She said that she would prefer to let the piece speak for itself.

The other two participants who had chosen the same phrase had written in very different ways. One had written a playful third person piece about being someone with a quicksilver personality who flitted about, changing focus frequently. The other wrote succinctly about feeling anxious about the future, and trying to stay in the present moment.

Another participant selected 'bitumen and pitch', which generated a sequence of words relating to a bereavement, carrying memories and feelings of anger and love. The writer cried whilst reading it out, and said later that he had felt a sense of release, both emotionally and through writing in a way that was much freer than he was used to.

The poem's opening line had resonated with a participant who wrote 'Where do I place my hope?' and conjured up a sense of bleakness through describing the absence of leaves on the trees. She gave a sharp rebuttal of irritating advice from others to 'think positive'. The piece ended with description of hopes for the future, and a sense of sadness and rage that these were being threatened.

The words 'borne hither and thither' led to a piece about sailing in a coracle over choppy waters, which for the writer represented the jokes and comments of people in a troublesome work environment which she was having difficulty negotiating.

One participant chose the phrase 'the way a body might put' and completed it with the words 'itself first, before the mind, and be kind'. This elicited responses from the group about how the body and mind can feel separate, and speculation about how a body could be 'kind' to its owner.

The activity took an hour and half, after which we had a tea break. A space had formed that was supportive and that would allow individuals opportunities for personal expression. People had been generous with written contributions and personal honesty. There had been laughter as well as tears.

I recognised afresh how organic the process can be, and how in each session like this I am a learner as well as facilitator, and feel both rewarded and humbled by this. I was left with an uplifting feeling that the group had its own positive momentum and that we could deepen and develop the work in exciting ways from here.

The Great Zoo   *Elaine Trevitt*

This is an exercise that came out of a Lapidus Scotland workshop, 'The Healing Power of Words / The Hurtful Power of Words', held over four days in the early autumn of 2004. We began by looking at the writing of blessings and curses and had gone on to explore the intersections of hurting and healing, of individual and group, of voice and listening, of work and play, of private and public.

Those present were poets and poetry therapists, writers with an interest in personal development, therapists with an interest in writing and others with varied experience on a continuum between writing and healing. We had been asked to do some preparatory work to get our hearts and minds into gear and to bring with us situations that were personally challenging and an openness to a community of fellow learners.

By the time The Great Zoo exercise was presented participants were generally feeling comfortable with each other and the atmosphere was supportive. There were five or six people with a facilitator in each of three groups for a reflective writing session that lasted about an hour and a quarter.

The Great Zoo is an exercise that has been used by writers as a means of exploring abstractions. The idea is taken from the Cuban poet, Nicolas Guillen (2004), who imagined the whole world to be a great zoo. Everything and anything can be in the zoo; the days of the week or the seasons; emotions, such as anger, jealousy or hope; bodily states, such as hunger or sleepiness; or indeed anything at all! The idea is to put the chosen concept, word or state into its own cage and to write a notice for it, as if it were an animal behind bars in a zoo. This is the notice that will enlighten the visitors. For example, in Guillen's own Great Zoo, a dream becomes a nocturnal butterfly, hunger is 'all fangs and eyes'.

Back to the exercise: what is it that you would put in your own zoo? Choose a 'creature'. Name it. What kind of creature is it? What is its natural habitat? What does it look like? What does it eat? Is it preyed upon or is it a predator? How does it reproduce? Is it nocturnal or diurnal? What is its temperament? What advice would you give to visitors? Remember to include a word of warning!

Using these prompts, write a notice that you would put up on your chosen creature's cage. Write in any way you wish but go with it fairly quickly, before too much thinking gets in the way. Guillen wrote poems; yours could be a poem, or it could be straightforward prose. Especially remember to include that word of warning.

The Wiston Lodge group added a nuance to the exercise. Given the emphasis of the workshop, that of exploring various intersections of opposites, and the general theme towards healing, it was not surprising that a spontaneous suggestion arose in one of the sub-groups that each person should choose two 'creatures', one 'negative' and one 'positive' attribute.

In what seemed like no time at all we had populated our own zoo. Here are some of the inhabitants:

Norma's creatures

Misery. Western variety. Lurks in muddy pools, well camouflaged, grabs passers-by as they get out of their depth. Jaws very strong, once gripped it is difficult to escape. Short sighted, doesn't like sunlight. Feeds on little doubts and fears.

Hope. Domestic specimen found in suburban environments, rural varieties increasingly rare. Beautiful singing voice, strong bones, little flesh.

Warning: do not expose to bad experiences. Keep warm and feed regularly with stories with happy endings.

Helen's creatures

Loneliness. Found at the poles and at high altitudes in lower latitudes; feeds on itself, hibernates diurnally and seasonally. Makes a low moaning sound which occasionally erupts into a shriek. Extremely fearful and timid; can bite when approached.

Resilience. Has a thick skin which it sheds and regrows annually. Will eat anything and adapt to any habitat. The female of the species outlives the male and is monogamous. Takes on average three mates and breeds four times over the course of a lifetime, but can thrive for long periods alone. Has survived numerous attempts at culling, and is known to live into its nineties.

Derek's creatures

Depression. This creature is slow and languorous and lives in dark places. He is, however, surprisingly resilient and persistent; when he corners his prey is loath to let go. He is especially difficult to shake off in the winter climates where he blends into the grey, toneless background. Beware of his teeth, they are sharper than you think.

Humour. This creature is quick moving and has a short attention span. It has bright colourful plumage and a distinctive call much like a kookaburra. It lives in warm welcoming environs and thrives in company. However, it can get vicious if given rough handling.

Glynis's creatures

Approach this sulk with extreme caution. It was captured in West Yorkshire and is believed to be around 50 years old. Do not prod nor use the expression 'better to have loved and lost'.

This enthusiasm is a shy creature and has not been seen in these parts for some time. Feel free to feed it. It is particularly fond of regular handfuls of hope and will respond well to praise. Please do not throw cold water on it.

Elaine's creatures

Disappointment. A creature often found exhausted after a long hard struggle. In captivity it requires a soft paddock with a bright outlook. Warning: if fed on bitter fruit, it may metamorphose into the more dangerous creature resentment.

Integrity. This creature is often found in difficult situations. It has an interesting habit of sticking its neck out when conditions become challenging but it is only dangerous to completely unrelated species. It is able to survive long periods of isolation but thrives best with a little companion.

The exercise was rated very highly by participants; it produced a lot of good humour and there was a neat finished product. It was felt that the pairings provided a nice balance between positive and negative attributes; if the writing was very personal it enabled a writer to see two sides to themselves. We discussed together how we might take it into another dimension by making a model zoo. It seemed there could be even more fun in arranging such a zoo spatially and that might also help clarify the relationships between the different 'creatures'. You would need to be careful not to place fragile hope next to enthusiasm, for instance, or it might get eaten up! And of course the exercise can be done without the pairings.

On 'Educating the Imagination'   *Dominic McLoughlin*

Perhaps when devising writing exercises, just as with writing poems, it is helpful to have a role model. Since I first read his book *I Never Told Anybody – Teaching Poetry Writing in a Nursing Home* (1977) my mentor in this way has been Kenneth Koch, the American poet and educator who died in 2002. The phrase 'educating the imagination' sums up Koch's approach and is the title of a key paper he gave to the Teachers and Writers Collaborative (1996, pp.153–67). Whilst he is not a bibliotherapist of any kind, it has been said that his approach encourages 'self-emancipation'. He was successful over many decades in encouraging children, patients and students all to write with a new-found joy in language. He inspired me to believe it was 'better to teach poetry writing as an art than to teach it – well, not really teach it but use it – as some form of distracting or consoling therapy' (1977, pp.43–4). I took this principle forward when working as a writer in hospices, prisons and other non-traditional educational settings.

The essence of Koch's approach is to trace the poems and ideas that got him excited about writing, and to think about how he learned from them. When advising other creative writing teachers he says, 'You're supposed to think the same things for yourself, you're not supposed to be so interested in what happened to me' (1996, p.157). From this I came to understand that learning and teaching is mainly being influenced, and allowing others to be influenced. To this end, for many years I developed a routine of bringing in a pair of poems to read and discuss as a prelude to writing in the workshop. The rationale for choosing a pair of poems in this way was that I valued how the two poems might be seen to work off each other and leave plenty of room for the reader to then take his own starting point from them. Examples of poems I brought together are Lavinia Greenlaw's 'From Scattered Blue' (1993, p.13) and Wordsworth's 'Composed upon Westminster Bridge' (1975, p.115); Sarah Maguire's 'No. 3 Greenhouse, 7.30 a.m.' (1997, p.36) and 'Come In' by Robert Frost (1971, p.195); and finally 'Mother, any distance greater than a single span' by Simon Armitage (1993, p.11) and Seamus Heaney's 'A Kite for Michael and Christopher' (1984, p.44). The pairings are made in an intuitive rather than a logical way. It is not that they share a form or a style. Rather that they can be shown to speak to one another in some way. This coupling mirrors something of the creative process itself (I think it was Paul Muldoon who said that writing a poem was always about bringing two ideas together to make a third thing).

I was lucky to have two valuable opportunities to work as a writer in health care, one at St Christopher's Hospice from 1991 to 1997 running a patients' writing group, and the other in an organisation providing residential care for men who were ex-offenders suffering with mental health problems. On many occasions in both settings I used this strategy of presenting the group with a pair of poems, then having some time to discuss them both independently and in relation to one another, and then setting a writing task that grew out of this. Sometimes I would have a clear idea of what the starting point for the writing exercise should be, but sometimes it flowed naturally out of our discussions of the poems in a way that I hadn't been able to see in advance. A recent example of a workshop run in this way is one I conducted as part of a short professional development course for writers in health and social care. The poems I took for students to look at were 'Apotheosis' by Jamie McKendrick (2003, p.1) and Sylvia Plath's 'The Arrival of the Bee Box' (1998, p.176). We read both the poems as a group. As a preamble to the discussion I would gauge participants' skills and interests in reading poetry, and address any concerns and preconceptions they might have. I did this because I didn't want anyone to feel excluded from discussion about poetry through lack of experience. I also like to harness any resistance people have towards it as a genre. As Ben Knights has shown (1995, pp.53–8) it is the difficulty of poetry that in part makes it valuable in a therapeutic setting.

On this occasion we had a good discussion about the two texts. But the way in to writing they indicated seemed hard to find. The other pairings that I mention above all seem to suggest something about poetry in general. For example they may allow us to think symbolically about poetry being a bridge, a threshold, or an anchor and a kite. McKendrick and Plath's bee poems seemed to go together, but I wanted to resist a reductive way in to writing ('Let's write about bees') because this sort of instruction is the last thing a writer wants to hear. It goes against the principle of 'educating the imagination', and Kenneth Koch suggests it would be likely to produce work that is empty and safe, rather than work that is – or has a chance of being – complex, serious and lyrical (1996, p.106). Thinking about this pair of poems subsequently I realise they are both, in their own way, about words. For me 'Apotheosis' is about the power of obsessive thinking, and shows we can get things out of proportion by holding forth on a single word or idea. The bee in this poem becomes huge and God-like. In 'The Arrival of the Bee Box' a jumble of bees interacts busily. Their movement suggests how words can become appalling, their noise like a kind of 'furious Latin'. In one workshop we found a starting point for writing, drawing on the idea of many and one. The students wrote fine poems about one a small thing happening in a big room, or a lots of things happening in a small room. Another way into writing reflecting the contrast in the two poems would be to present participants with a single word, and a list of say ten words randomly chosen. The writing task could be to write a poem either out of the group of words or inspired by just one.

Edges, Risks and Connections: Reflections on a Workshop Led by John Fox   *Leone Ridsdale*

From the top of the bus on the way there I saw flags of St George waving disconsolately from cars, remnants of the World Cup. At Notting Hill Gate, I turned down quiet Palace Gardens, until I came to number 104. John came to the door, and led me to a group sitting in a circle in the middle of a church. John told us about his life. Long stays in orthopaedic hospitals had marked his childhood, and ended in the loss of his leg. He recounted how writing and facilitating writing had been a therapeutic process for him. He then led us on imperceptibly to an exercise. It may have started with a meditation which, in a church, did not seem out of place. He had given us a book of poems, sayings and stories that were important to him. He started reading. A child aged eight had written an anthem called 'If you praise a word, it turns into a poem'. I have little experience of poetry beyond school. Continuing in my thoughts I wrote:

> I am like a speck of dust,
>   it can be seen vibrating
> The sun beats down
> There is a shaft of shade,
>   and dust can be seen dancing.
> I am here moving,
>   vulnerable and evanescent...

The next exercise was stimulated by a poem John had written himself called 'When someone deeply listens to you'. He read it, and sometimes looked up at us, saying it by heart. He asked us to use the first line to begin writing about ourselves. A member of the group wrote:

Listening by Alison Clayburn

> When you listen to me deeply
> I grow lighter.
> My edges meet the air,
> the ice coat drops away
> and I rise.
>
> When I listen to you deeply
> I grow larger.
> A soft and heavy largeness forms,
> then settles comfortably
> against the earth.

I wrote:

> When someone deeply listens to me
> I feel understood.

I make connections
between my life now and my life then...

When someone deeply listens to me
and simply repeats back something I have said,
suddenly I resonate with the emotion that I experienced
before.
It catches me unexpectedly.
Sometimes I stop and feel it breaking across me like a wave,
the sadness, the anger, sometimes it's too much.
I feel my throat tightening as I speak,
and try to carry myself forward
by talking, to something else...

At lunch we filed out into the sunshine, bought sandwiches and ate them in the gardens of the church. It was autumn, and a little cold, but it was an opportunity to talk. It seemed natural that after lunch we moved into a smaller room where we could hear each other more easily, and start by saying a bit about ourselves.

The afternoon seemed short, but I noticed that when people read John listened attentively. He sometimes sighed and breathed as though his body was in tune with the voice he listened to and the message. Afterwards there was a silence, and he would ask the reader to read it again. The process was deeply respectful and valuing. It heard and allowed each person to express her own truth. People read and said how they felt about their own experiences, and I resonated too.

The last exercise was stimulated by a poem about a man coming to terms with his wife's cancer. John picked words from the poem, 'I don't know...', and asked us to do the final exercise. I wrote:

I don't know
what's wrong with you
You want me to know,
know now, help, do something

I feel this urgency
It makes me tense
this neediness in you

I don't know
what's wrong with you
It may take a long time

And when I do know
I may not be able to help
I may not be able to do something

I do want to know,
know now,
help,
do something

It's just not possible.

I feel your stress, your distress
I am stressed and distressed

But I must move on now
We must go to see the next patient

I was surprised in reading this out how much it disturbed me, a normal aspect of my life as a doctor. Not knowing, enquiring, and then moving towards some provisional knowing is usual, but also fraught.

A member of the group, Alison Clayburn, wrote:

The work of fire and hands
I don't know what
will make this arrow work, wing
its way upward, turn
into a firework, scatter
sparkles for miles around.
I don't know how
to protect it from the rainstorms
of looks from strangers,
blaring microphones and plasma screens
that seem to want it to be nothing
but a damp stub hiding
in my plastic ego, waiting

  for a boot heel to grind it
  into the gravel, for a hand to lift it
  and place it in a skip...

Soon we were leaving. It was a good group. I enjoyed the day and learned. Reading, writing and reading can be a therapeutic and transforming process. I do not know how much more might be achieved if this workshop had been for longer than a day, and wonder if the process was itself poetry.

CHAPTER 5

Writing in Form

Edited by Victoria Field

There is a paradox in life that sometimes having too much choice can make it impossible to take a decision. In therapeutic writing situations, we often say there are no rules and constraints, and that whatever the writer wants to write is valid. This is true on one level and an absence of any 'right or wrong' in writing is one of the stated *sine qua non*s of writing therapeutically. However, the freedom to 'just write' can also be unhelpful, especially to people who are new to this approach. Sometimes constraints, parameters or suggestions can make the task of writing more, rather than less, accessible. In Chapter 1, Kate Thompson introduced techniques where participants are given small, manageable writing suggestions to get over that barrier. In this chapter, four contributors show how a more extended exploration of specific forms in poetry can have therapeutic benefits and, finally, suggestions are made for a kind of 'writing in form' for prose: genre writing.

The use of form and especially rhyme in poetry can be a surprisingly hot issue in writing groups. It may be seen as exclusive and elitist, particularly by people who have unhappy memories of formal education. For others, form or rhyme can appear to obscure or even prevent deeper thought and be old fashioned or unsophisticated – perhaps like figurative painting. Conversely, some people find the perceived formlessness of modern poetry a case of the 'emperor's new clothes' and welcome structure as evidence of an ability to craft words. These different views struck me forcefully some years ago. In a beautiful spring week, I used Wordsworth's 'Daffodils' with a group of hospital patients who responded warmly and enthusiastically, creating a group poem in response. I then took the same poem to a group at a day treatment and therapy centre, the members of which had been writing their own poetry for some time. There, it was derided as an example of pompous poetic posturing! The latter response came as a complete surprise to me; it subsequently led to very useful discussions of what it means to write authentically, however, and how those individuals felt vis-à-vis a perceived poetry 'establishment'.

Two very practical books on writing poetry, which focus on contemporary poets whilst still exploring structural matters such as metre and form, are *Writing Poems* by Peter Sansom (1994) and *Teach Yourself Writing Poetry* by John Hartley Williams and Matthew Sweeney (1997): all three of whom are celebrated contemporary poets.

The reason for suggesting writing in given forms is usually that it paradoxically frees the writer. As he or she focuses on technicalities such as metre or end-rhyme, the unconscious is simultaneously finding the appropriate image or metaphor. This can be analogous to seeing a dim star more clearly whilst not looking straight at it. Gillie Bolton describes the use of haiku especially to encourage an engagement with the natural world. Its basic rule of three lines, 17 syllables, makes it a particularly unthreatening form for new-comers to writing; although I have always enjoyed a haiku attributed to John Cooper Clarke which says:

> Expressing yourself
> in seventeen syllables
> is very diffi.

It is a form which everyone, including young children, can attempt to their own satisfaction.

Kennings, which like haiku are now taught in school, are pairings of nouns to describe a familiar object in a new way. They were common in Old English and Old Norse poetry – where the sea can be called the 'whale-road', and a battle, a 'storm of swords'. Thus, a chair can become a 'bottom-supporter', a rabbit, a 'carrot-cruncher'. I have asked groups to suggest kennings for, for example, 'mother'. Doing this as a group exercise can make it playful and non-threatening. Kennings that emerged included: cake-creator, milk-withholder, worry-machine, lip-purser, bosom-snuggler, moment-spoiler and so on. Individuals then used these phrases either to make a poem composed of kennings or as a jumping off point for a different piece of writing.

Repetition is a hallmark of poetry. A chorus or refrain repeats a whole stanza. Forms such as the villanelle repeat lines; a sestina repeats words at the end of lines; rhyme, assonance and alliteration repeat sounds. Kate Thompson here describes using pantoums – in which lines are repeated –

to encourage journal writers to try poetry. Her step-by-step approach is a model of how to set up a task so that those trying it for the first time will be able to succeed. It is important when introducing poetic form in a therapeutic writing setting that everyone can participate: failing or 'not getting it' can reinforce a sense of inadequacy.

Sonnets are a difficult form and there are more and less constraining variants. Robert Hamberger describes how it is this very difficulty that enables him to write about the most emotive topics. Robert Frost has famously described writing free verse as being 'like playing tennis with the net down' (Frost 1935). Here Robert Hamberger describes how putting the net higher and higher gives him a sense of security when writing on sensitive topics. This is one approach and appropriate for an experienced poet. I have argued for subverting or loosening forms to make a bridge between them and free verse – for example, a 'sort-of sonnet' that:

> honours the shape of the thought and poetic tradition but does not insist on the matching gloves, shoes and handbag of an earlier time. That there is pleasure in a perceived pattern that isn't saying 'look at me' at the expense of my content... (Field 2004a, p.10)

The tension between freedom and control, spontaneity and measured reflection is inherent in all writing practice. Usually, in a therapeutic setting, spontaneity is prioritised, whilst in writing for publication, control and measured reflection are vital.

A very basic use of form is simple rhyming. Children love rhyme and, for adults too, its incantatory, nonsense or nursery qualities can help us tap into emotions very directly and often unconsciously. Subverting nursery rhymes, writing in ballad form or creating new song lyrics for favourite tunes all require finding rhymes. As Robert Hamberger describes, sometimes what at first might seem a forced or inappropriate rhyme can lead to new insights.

Jane Tozer also chooses a difficult form to write about a deeply personal experience. Her moving account of writing a ghazal shows how, even for an experienced poet, an encounter with a completely new form, unfamiliar in Western culture, enabled her to move into a different kind of sensibility.

Finally, Gillie Bolton discusses the use of genre writing. Here, rather than the choice of words being restricted (as in the use of poetic form), the choice of character and setting is restricted in order to conform with (or sometimes subvert) the stereotypical or 'stock' characters and settings of various narrative genres. Once again, the restrictions paradoxically free the writer – the use of settings such as a forest, a palace, a spaceship or even an idealised hospital, which are far from the usual milieu of the writer, can sometimes create a safe space where deeper emotional truths can be explored.

Haiku   *Gillie Bolton*

up from the valley
gold larch needles edge the lane
stitching back my heart (Bolton 1999, p.41)

This tiny poem has 17 syllables set out in a specific form, expressing an intense moment of experience. Through close attention to humble and everyday natural details a haiku writer (and reader) can experience profoundly held truths of life. Description of the object is not enough. Haiku writers do not look *at* but *as* the aspect of nature about which they are writing: 'Learn about a pine tree from a pine tree… The poet enters into the object, sharing its delicate life and its feelings. Whereupon a poem forms itself', as the great fifteenth-century Japanese haiku master Basho taught (Stryk 1985, p.14).

The philosophy behind haiku says that in losing oneself in involvement with the natural world, the writer becomes open to learning everything of importance, thereby open to gaining peace and acceptance of life's vicissitudes.

Health and fitness gurus exhort people to go out, breathe deeply and feel part of nature. It's well known that contemplation of the night sky can ease depression and anxiety, for example. Haiku takes this two steps further. The first is that it asks one not only to absorb a sense of nature into the self, but to absorb the self into nature. The next step is to express that experience, the 'haiku moment', in writing. The process of expression, succinctly, simply and joyously, deepens insight and clarity about the self, and closeness to and understanding of nature.

Haiku, a traditional Japanese form since the eighth century, were of course expressed in characters. As Japanese is a language without stresses, unlike English, syllable counting is more straightforward when there is no possibility of iambics (the de-dum rhythm of Shakespeare and Wordsworth), or any other metre. English haiku therefore is an adaptation of the form. Syllable counting and line length are not the most important elements of haiku. If a tiny poem does not express a 'haiku moment' it is not a haiku, however accurate the counting.

Haiku encourages a dwelling in the now, an awareness that the kingdom of heaven is at hand, if you like. It prevents anxiously anticipating the future, or dwelling in the past. The present is all we have, yet many miss it by concentrating on what may never be, or on what cannot be changed because it is done and past. We only have one life: there is no rehearsal, no debrief. This can lead to a fuller appreciation of and respect for ordinary everyday life.

How to write haiku

A mood of stillness needs to be fostered. Writers calmly allow their minds to focus upon a detail. It is the allowing of the natural world to speak through the poem, rather than a conscious focusing, which makes it a haiku.

Then the image is expressed in a very concise way (the *Oxford English Dictionary* gives one meaning of 'concise' as being to put a silk band around something). Formal Haiku have 17 syllables: five in the first line, seven in the second and five in the third. One tiny image of nature is evoked; wider implications are left to the reader's imagination.

This poem of mine is not really a haiku because of its metaphorical and punning artifice:

> in a depression
> of rock after heavy rain
> a clear pool settles

My 'larch needles' at the beginning of this section is nearer, but it is unsubtly too clear what I am getting at ('stitching back my heart'). Though I think Basho does also to an extent sometimes tell the reader:

> Sparrows in eaves
> mice in ceiling –
> celestial music (1985, p.27 Stryk[1])

---

[1]   'Sparrow in eaves' (p.14) from *On Love and Barley: Haiku of Basho* by Basho, translated with an introduction by Lucien Stryk (Penguin Classics, 1985). Copyright © Lucien Stryk, 1985. Reproduced by permission of Penguin Books Ltd.

I received an anonymous e-mail years ago telling me that in Japan they have replaced impersonal and unhelpful computer error messages with haiku-like poetry messages, such as:

> Chaos reigns within
> Reflect, repent, and reboot
> Order shall return

> Yesterday it worked
> Today it is not working
> Windows is like that

> With searching comes loss
> And the presence of absence:
> 'My Novel' not found.

Renga traditionally are linked haiku, originally written by two people: linked verses rather than a narrative. In Japan there are frequent renga parties where poetry writing is alive and well and an integral part of life. I have used the form in threes. Everyone writes a haiku-like poem on a piece of paper and passes it on to the person on their left. They then all write another one linked to the first. The papers are passed on again for a third poem to be written on each paper. This can be introduced as thesis, antithesis and synthesis, or just as a linked threesome. The trios are read out in turn, the final writer reading the three on the paper on which they wrote the last haiku. Here are a pair written at the end of a week-long healing writing retreat:

> Window glass and mist
> between me and the beeches,
> candle's heat shakes them (Gillie Bolton)

> Candle is blown out
> the wind's breath waves the beeches
> I watch the mist lift (Diana King)

Pantoums   *Kate Thompson*

In journal writing groups there can be resistance to the suggestion of writing poetry (see AlphaPoems in Chapter 1). Members' prejudices can range from 'I can't be a poet, I'm not a man/dead/good enough' or 'I'm not clever enough to understand poems' to 'I hate poetry' or 'poetry is boring' stemming from bad experiences at school, feelings of inadequacy or simply exposure to bad or boring poetry.

Anthony Burgess (1986) makes a distinction between pianists, who are professional, talented musicians, and piano-players, who are people whose enjoyment lies in playing for themselves or others but who have no pretension to a higher reputation or public acclaim. In journal writing groups or other groups writing for personal development, it is perhaps useful to make a similar distinction between poem-making and writing poetry (or poem-makers and poets). This allows participants to give themselves permission to play and enjoy the activity for its own sake without feeling inadequate or unable to meet some perceived standards. It does not preclude a poet emerging, or a poem-maker writing a good poem, but it does give enjoyment a higher priority than art.

The more rigid the form the easier it is to guide people into the writing of poems. Rules and structure give people confidence to attempt something new by breaking the experience down into small, manageable steps or tasks. This approach also provides containment for the rising anxiety of 'Am I doing it right? What should I do next?'

A pantoum is an ancient Indonesian verse form with 16 lines in four stanzas with only eight different lines. The circularity of the form makes it ideal for journal writing and reflection. This form offers an ideal example of poem-making which can help overturn those prejudices with surprising results. Because it builds up gradually people suddenly find they have a poem before they realise it; the process of working at line level allows the whole poem to emerge unobserved and therefore uncensored. It's like walking up a steep path, concentrating on each step, then turning round and seeing the whole landscape. Facilitators lead participants step by step to the whole poem.

The Creative Journal Group met for a term in the 'Personal Development' section of the adult education service. The 12 registered names became nine physical bodies whose reasons for being there ranged from 'I've always wanted to write' to 'I always do a new course in the spring' and 'I get bored with writing about who I've met in my diary'. From this diverse collection emerged a group which supported each other through various emotional issues and who continued to meet to write long after the course was over.

Donna, the youngest member of the Creative Journal Group, was studying for her A levels at the local college and still suffering from a surfeit of GCSE poetry; she joined the group six months after her mother's death. Janet, the oldest member of the group, could still remember being force-fed a diet of Victorian patriotic verse to be learnt by heart. She almost left the group at the idea of writing poetry and I could feel the waves of scepticism, mixed with fear, emanating from her. Nevertheless, pantoums it was.

I had begun the session by guiding people to write a Captured Moment from the past week, something which stood out from the week richer in emotional memory than surrounding times and which they would fill with as much sensory detail as they could (Adams 1990: see Chapter 7). I then asked people to select a line or phrase from their Captured Moment which resonated or intrigued them.

'That's your first line,' I said. 'All I want you to do is write three more lines to follow it, just four lines of verse. It doesn't have to rhyme.'

Gradually I saw them all uncurling their resistance and connecting with their writing again, reluctantly at first but then, when their confidence grew, with more conviction. Vera looked almost smug; she had previously written verse for greeting cards – she could rhyme with a vengeance.

'The next stanza begins with the second line you wrote. Now a new line; now Line 4 from the first stanza; now a new line. That's your second stanza.'

Fear receded, brows cleared: they now had two complete stanzas each.

'Stanza 3 consists of two repeated lines alternated with new lines: 5–7–6–8. Your final stanza is a reprise of lines: 7–3–8–1. That's it, you've done it.'

'It does look rather like a poem,' Janet murmured tentatively.
Donna wrote:

I sit at the kitchen table	1
Christmases past in its grain	2
Mind full of fairy lights of childhood	3
And my mother's welcoming smile	4
Christmases past in its grain	2
The table remembers it all	5
And my mother's welcoming smile	4
Lighting up the familiar room	6
The table remembers it all	5

My brother and I snapping crackers	7
Lighting up the familiar room	6
Echoing gaiety now gone	8
My brother and I snapping crackers	7
Mind full of fairy lights of childhood	3
Echoing with with gaiety now gone	8
I sit at the kitchen table	1

We read them out and even Janet grudgingly admitted that they were just about poems and she had created one of her own which she might not disown. Vera said it was quite liberating not to have to rhyme every time.

Why Sonnets?   *Robert Hamberger*

I shamefacedly admit that I've written sonnets since I was a bookish teenager. Why the attraction? At that time, writing sonnets was a challenging puzzle. Could I finish 14 lines, with end-rhymes in a fixed pattern, that still made sense and retained my voice? As a teenager I failed; but having now written 80 or more sonnets, the balancing act of puzzle and creativity – order and fluidity – remains to drag me back to that form.

One of Edna St Vincent Millay's late sonnets sums up the tension and attraction when she writes:

> I will put Chaos into fourteen lines
> And keep him there. (1988, p.153)

The moment I read those lines in a bookshop, I knew that she understood why I'm repeatedly drawn to sonnets. The start of any poem is wordlessness struggling for voice, a rhythm and shape, a temporary break from silence. In the early drafting process, when a poem starts to nudge itself towards the sonnet form, I know that the tussle of finding the right rhymes and half-rhymes, in the expected order, will give me a template in which the mess of my emotions might temporarily feel secure enough to speak. Imagination is subversive. It's as if the editing part of the mind is so distracted by hunting the next rhyme that it allows the saboteur – the rule-breaker – to smuggle taboo words under the apparent barbed-wire of form.

Fifteen years ago I wrote a sequence called 'Acts of Parting'. It was basically about my experience during the last illness of my best friend

Clifford, whom I'd known since we met as 11-year-olds on our first
morning at secondary school. When I write a sequence of poems, in each
case it doesn't begin with a calculated decision, which I plot like a military
campaign. There's usually a gradual realisation that a cluster of themes is
insisting on more space and attention than one poem will permit. So the
possibility of a sequence, and (in the process of writing) the shape that each
sequence insists on, evolves.

With 'Acts of Parting' I knew instinctively, after writing the first three
free-verse poems, that I wanted free-verse to alternate with sonnets.
Obviously, when starting the sequence, I couldn't foresee that the next six
months would carry us all through Clifford's last illness. He had contracted
HIV five years before, and in those days combination therapies to manage
the condition were at a relatively early stage. So, while my conscious mind
was willing him back to health, and my days were filled with hospital and
home visits, supporting his partner and mother, juggling the needs of my
wife and young children, keeping my job and house going, I understood
that I needed the space to find words for what I was experiencing.

It appeared to be a mixture of instinct and conscious choice when I
deliberately picked the Petrarchan form for the 'Acts of Parting' sonnets. I
view this as the strictest sonnet form, because it only allows the poet four
rhymes (compared to Shakespearean sonnets with seven rhymes). It felt as
if I was choosing a form whereby the apparent straitjacket of a limited
rhyme-scheme would hold me tight, give me a strange sense of security.
There's no doubt that my emotions at the time were wild, contradictory
and apparently incoherent. How could I give them words, allow them to
speak?

As I recall, the sonnets came slowly, but they were written during the
immediacy of my experience. This was far from Wordsworth's
recommendation of emotion recollected in tranquillity. But at the same
time writing those sonnets promised the relative safety of an empty page, a
quiet space to confront my experience as honestly as possible. One poem I
wrote at this time describes the simultaneously wonderful and tortured
period of remission during a long and difficult terminal illness:

Remission *by Robert Hamberger*

Now you know they can do nothing for you
you go home, walking out of hospital

as if walking is one of those beautiful
humdrum acts you reclaim, like standing in a queue
or using your own key. You're back in charge for two
months, ten, twenty. Anything's possible
when you talk like that. Risk it: be hopeful.
For weeks we watched a hyena chew
your fat, skinning you to the bone. Scratching a flea
it yawns and drops you now. It will let
you walk away for a while, plotting to be free:
'Listen. We'll go to London and send that
fucking doctor a photo of me
in a kiss-me-quick hat saying Not Dead Yet.'
(Hamberger 1997, p.51)

I remember the first line being a stark admission to myself at the time: they can do nothing for him. I was almost saying to myself *Face it* when that line stared back at me from the page. Writing sonnets usually includes the poet scribbling lists of 'nose blows rose', as Don Paterson describes that undignified scramble for the right rhyme (Paterson 1999, p.xxii), or (often, in my case) half-rhyme. Rhyming pushes a poet to examine both the music and meaning of a limited list of words, the possibilities of which can tip a poet towards images they hadn't previously imagined or expected. This is how the hyena arrived halfway through the sonnet, apparently out of nowhere: simply because chew rhymed with two, queue and you. What creature or process might chew in this context; how could chew fit into this poem, or should I discard it for another rhyme? Hooking onto that rhyme led to the horrible recognition of what we'd been watching during Clifford's last illness, and how he was escaping for a while. All poetry can (and perhaps should) jolt a poet during its composition, but rhyme is certainly another trick for catching a poet unawares, surprising their controls by the accuracy of a metaphor or image they may otherwise have ignored.

It seems no coincidence that Dylan Thomas (an often freewheeling poet in relation to form) chose the rigorous rules of a villanelle for 'Do Not Go Gentle into That Good Night' (1998), as if its discipline could hold his grief in check for long enough to address his dying father. In the process he achieved one of the finest examples of that apparently artificial form.

It's equally significant that Gerard Manley Hopkins' six sonnets (1953), usually known as the Terrible Sonnets for their painful subject matter, express spiritual desolation in an acutely personal way, yet each are held tight within the Petrarchan form. His biographer Robert Bernard Martin explains the paradox of these poems with a:

> sense of contained anarchy, of inchoate, almost unspeakable emotion given verbal form… Whether or not he thought out the matter, the fact is that [Hopkins] chose one of the most disciplined verse forms because it best held his explosive emotions in check. These poems shock doubly because of the contrast between the decorum of the sonnet form and the dark energy pulsing against its restraints. (Martin 1991, p.383)

The continued popularity of the sonnet for love poetry since its origins in thirteenth-century Italy may partly be explained by the fact that falling in love is itself a period of extreme emotion, akin perhaps to a sense of chaos in relation to the former self. So the sonnet's semblance of direction lends a steadying hand through the blind alleys and happy accidents of composition. Don Paterson said, 'Poets write sonnets because it makes poems easier to write' (1999, p.xxii). The paradox is that strict form can, at times, become a liberation, an odd permission for the poet to allow their saboteur (their chaotic emotions) to speak plainly. If you're lucky, and during the drafting process your words and images coalesce into an order that both surprises you and confirms your truth-telling instincts, the sonnet will give shape to:

> nothing more nor less
> Than something simple not yet understood.
> (St Vincent Millay 1988, p.153)

Ghazal: A Poem of Love and Loss   *Jane Tozer*

My story

The cause of my (moderately severe) depression lies in a dire happening at university when I was 19. Having been helped by cognitive therapy, I can speak of this experience. But it remains a painful subject, and I'm still unable to write about it. Childlessness, too, is a protracted heartache. Perhaps I never will be able to express these things in poetry; they are more five-act tragedy than ghazal. Perhaps I don't need to write about them.

My mum was ignorant of the circumstances. She always blamed my sporadic bouts of depression on the lost love of my youth. He was a brilliant student, whom I met while I was teaching English in Finland, 1970–71. We were soul-mates, beautiful, gifted, utterly in love, frighteningly vulnerable. He was 17, I was 21. In those days, such an age difference was transgressive. When my year's contract ran out, I came back to Britain. We were 1200 miles apart, under a cloud of parental disapproval, penniless and striving for the freedom to be together.

In 1972, aged 22, I had my first breakdown, triggered by teaching practice in a tough Yorkshire school. By the time I recovered from anxiety and depression, it was too late for me to go back to Finland. It took decades to regain confidence in my poetic voice.

In 2003, after nearly 30 years' silence, I found him via the internet. He is, like me, happily married. We are in occasional cheerful contact by phone and e-mail. This rediscovery unlocked a compartment in my unconscious, the box with his name on it. It was, and remains, an obsession, but it has become a creative one.

What ghazal did for me

In writing a ghazal, I found a lost register of my poetic voice, and zapped a monstrous writer's block. Until that day, I'd been reticent about myself in my poems; I've always dreaded lapsing into sentimentality and making an arse of myself. Poetic forms allow control over just how much self we expose, rather than letting it all hang out. The ghazal form connected me with intensely personal subject matter.

Poetry often works paradoxically. For me, the most exhilarating paradox is that rules can be liberating. When writing in traditional formal structures, the trick is to forget the imagined teacher-in-your-head, who values conformity more than originality. Poetic form is the foundation on which you build, but remember that you are the architect, and you are not building a prison.

Ghazal history and form

Interest in the ghazal was aroused in the USA by the Kashmiri-American poet Agha Shahid Ali (1949–2001). He is ghazal's most famous modern exponent, an acknowledged master. In the UK, the ghazal has a passionate and inspiring advocate in the Iranian-born British poet Mimi Khalvati. It is a traditional form with origins in the old Persian empire and neighbouring Islamic cultures and has complex conventions. The best way to get information is by an internet search.

Some of its many conventions are as follows:

- It has 5–15 couplets. There is never an enjambment (run-on) between the couplets.

- Think of each couplet as a separate poem – like a pearl on a string: lovely in its own right, even more lustrous among other pearls. Line 2 should amplify Line 1, turning things around, surprising us.

- The couplets are linked by a strict formal scheme, centred on a refrain (radif). The structure may be further enriched by rhyme. Each line must be of the same length (inclusive of the refrain and/or rhyme).

- The last couplet is usually a signature couplet in which the poet invokes their name in the first, second or third person. It's easier in languages where names have identifiable meaning.

- There is an epigrammatic terseness in the ghazal, but with immense lyricism, evocation, sorrow, heartbreak, wit. What defines the ghazal is a constant longing.

Writing my ghazal

In 2003, Mimi Khalvati tutored a poetry workshop in Cornwall. She challenged us to write a ghazal in under an hour, suggesting that the form enabled the poet to write with more personal emotion than is fashionable in modern Western poetry. It might help us to walk closer to the edge of sentimentality and create lines of genuine beauty. An apparently gentle, fragile poem may pack a big punch. In ghazal, unfulfilled desire may be used wittily, to make all kinds of political, social, moral, satirical points.

My eureka moment came when Mimi explained that 'ghazal' and 'gazelle' have the same etymology. The tone of ghazal is the cry of the wounded deer. Faiz Ahmed Faiz believed that the true subject of lyric poetry was the loss of the beloved. Longing for the beloved is conflated with longing for the divine. However, this longing is not platonic; the beloved is very much flesh and blood.

This was synchronicity of the spookiest kind; the gazelle's cry echoed the obsession of my heart. My back-story of lost love meant that I came to the exercise with ready-made subject, imagery, location, colour, tone, music. I spent an absorbed 50 minutes in a sunny garden; it seemed a very Persian thing to do. The ghazal emerged complete, needing only minor cuts.

Having recently translated a book-length mediaeval poem in rhyming couplets, my ear was tuned in to rhyme and metre. The rhythm I use gives the lines a Border Ballad-like effect. There is a central caesura in each line; this poise between the two halves of the line recalls Finnish folk poetry and the epic 'Kalevala'. So, counter to tradition, my ghazal does have a fragmentary narrative structure.

It uses the European convention of the end-rhymed couplet. Or rather, in this case, half-rhymed assonant couplet. When I wrote it, I wasn't even aware that silver is one of those words which famously has no true rhyme.

Ghazal in Silver

In Finnish, the first syllable is always stressed. 'Sau' in 'sauna' rhymes with 'how now, brown cow'.

A few stilted snapshots, like bent tarnished silver.
    I am reading your letters. A miser counts silver.

Kultani, my gold, means sweetheart, my lover –
    I still feel your skin with its soft bloom of silver.

After *sauna*, we swim in the lake's cool grey water
    And the swans twine their necks of exquisite silver.

I was your first, and you – my soul's brother;
    Incongruous metals, fierce steel and soft silver.

The words lovers long for are *always* and *never.*
    What runs through their veins is the purest quicksilver.

Each planted a birch. Now their branches arch over.
    No tree in England is so clear a silver.

Down at the dockside, we're limbs torn asunder
    Stand howling like wolves in the moon's snowy silver.

Your ship slips its mooring and slides down the river.
    My tears clatter down like a handful of silver.

My mother blamed you. We were parted forever.
    She earned no forgiveness till her hair turned silver.

A lake, and storks calling. Sibelius shiver.
  Their note stretches, breaks. It is colder than silver.

The lovers in stories are brother and sister.
  The warlords sell guns, and their bullets are silver.

Genre   *Gillie Bolton*

Genre is when a recognisable form of characterisation, plot structure, situation and time scale is used: fairy story ('Once upon a time there was a wise wizard…'); sugary romance ('"Oh!" she sighed as she fell into his arms…'); detective ('"Aha," she said. "So it WAS you!"'); fantasy ('The angel opened a door in the sky; I stepped through after him…'); thriller ('She paused, heart pounding, listening to the approaching footsteps'); soap opera ('I'm just putting the kettle on, want a coffee?'); specific forms of poetry (pastiche can be very funny: 'My love is like a hot rotting compost heap'); sci-fi (the space ship with a human heart) – and so on…

I have asked medical and health-care clinicians, children, teachers and those in training for therapeutic writing to write such stories and poems. Genre writing can be very illuminative as the writer does not have to bother with characterisation – all the characters are *flat* archetypes (wizards; sleuths; farmers; tall, dark and impossibly handsome strangers). And the situations depicted can be equally undemanding to conjure up (behind the hayrick, in the pub, a churchyard on a dark night, a cave in the centre of a huge whispering wood).

Writers pick images and characters and settings off the peg from their own version of our culture (the woodcutter's daughter being kissed in the castle by a frog who turns into a pumpkin). They use such stock characters and situations to explore whatever they need to explore. Little Red Riding Hood or Sleeping Beauty have been depicted as victims of incest for example. This is an area for which genre writing is extremely illuminative, although it needs careful handling, of course (for more information see Bolton 2003). The power of the results can be astonishing: both to writers themselves and to their readers. The only time I remember it not working was when a nurse really wanted to explore gender issues in nursing. She did not succeed in writing a romantic love story with a woman doctor and a male nurse, however hard she tried. Perhaps she might have succeeded if both doctor and nurse had been female.

The conclusion to *Writing Works* includes examples of genre stories by both Gillie and Kate in which they use the conventions of a fairy story to explore their own journeys in the field of therapeutic writing.

PART TWO

Writing from Within

CHAPTER 6

What People Need to Write

Edited by Kate Thompson

A theme of this chapter is trust, trust at many different levels. Dominique De-Light says 'Trust is key'. Of course none of the exercises or examples in this book would work without trust between the facilitator and the group or client. The relationship is therefore of great significance and it works both ways. In several of the exercises below, authors describe how people write what they want to write and what they need to write, all of which require a degree of trust of each other and of the self.

In her piece Jeannie Wright's 'tutor persona' trusts her group enough to be able to do the exercise herself and to be engaged enough for the process to produce surprisingly authentic results; indeed, she allows herself to be shaken by what she writes. It is often a question of debate as to whether the facilitator should herself write during the sessions and if so whether to share her writing with the group. My own experience has been that groups do like their facilitator to join in but there are times when this would clearly not be appropriate. The challenge is to be present but not self-absorbed. The role of the facilitator is as varied as the needs of the group and the complexity of the exercise.

Therapeutic writing can often have surprising outcomes (Lindy in Kate Evans' piece expressing her anger), unforeseen benefits (Dominique De-Light mentions how writing had led to behaviour change for several participants; Kathleen Adams' client managed to make life changes after her writing) and unexpected revelations (Maria Antoniou explores the story of a missing twin in family stories and Maeve in Fiona Hamilton's piece discovers her childlike self again) but these can also bring up painful or disturbing material. Maria Antoniou suggests that her exercise should be conducted by an experienced facilitator for this very reason. In this chapter, as in others, we find examples of 'Aha' moments, moments we greet with recognition, when things suddenly fall into place, when we have a new insight.

Trusting the process and trusting the self are recurring themes both here and in other sections. Fiona Hamilton writes of needing to 'plan less and trust more' in order to allow the writing to emerge in the moment. She works to be fully present with Maeve by actively listening on different levels.

The genesis of Maria Antoniou's exercise was a piece of personal writing which she felt compelled to write. She demonstrates that inspiration can strike at any time and that it is worth remembering that what works for us can be useful for others in a variety of guises.

Kathleen Adams has developed a technique based on trilogies where each stage takes the writer further down to the material which needs to be expressed. She tells us how this technique can start from any of the familiar exercises we use.

Writing can be therapeutic whether or not that is made explicit and intentional. For some people, perhaps because of their previous experiences in the mental health services, the word 'therapeutic' might alienate many clients even though those are the benefits they are seeking, as Dominique De-Light points out. The variety of exercises and the way that they are presented may determine what people write to some extent but they are merely a vehicle for people to use if they wish. The beneficial result is produced by people writing what they need to write and perhaps the facilitator's role is really to enable this.

Series of Three   *Kathleen Adams*

The world abounds in natural trilogies: yesterday, today, tomorrow. Inside, outside, centre. Birth, death, rebirth. Maiden, mother, crone. High, low, middle. Body, mind, spirit. Plant, bloom, wither. We, you, they. Good, bad, indifferent.

Journal therapy is no exception. A trilogy of writes – a Series of Three – can identify, clarify, resolve.

The Series of Three is three consecutive writes, using the same technique, each building on the one before it. When the second and third writes are intentionally and mindfully taken from the write that preceded it, the layering can have a remarkably healing or useful effect.

Sophie came to session with a powerful hurt and anger at her boss, who belittled her in meetings, took credit for her ideas and made her feel small and insignificant. 'I lose all my personal power around him!' she complained.

'What do you want to be able to say to him?' I queried.

She listed a litany of complaints. 'But it's useless,' she said. 'I've tried to talk to him a half-dozen times. I have written polite memos, I've had assertive, reasonable conversations. Nothing changes. Maybe I should quit!'

'Maybe so,' I said. 'But before you do, let's try some journal work. Write an Unsent Letter. Write as hard and fast as you can. Don't hold back. Don't be polite or reasonable. Just say exactly how you feel. This isn't leaving your journal.'

For ten minutes, I watched as Sophie's pen flew. Her writing became enlarged and erratic. She wasn't staying neatly on the lines. Faster and faster she wrote, with deepened pressure. When I called time, she signed her name with a flourish.

I pulled an empty chair around to face her. 'Read it out loud,' I said. 'Imagine Mr Bad Boss sitting in that chair, with a piece of tape over his mouth. He can't answer back. It's all about you.'

Sophie chuckled. She stared hard at the chair, then dropped her eyes and began to read from her page. When she finished, I motioned her over to the empty chair.

'Now, if you're willing, I'd like you to move over here to this chair and "become" Mr Bad Boss. He has something he wants to say in response to your letter. It's his turn to have all the stage. He's going to write about what's really going on for him, not what he says out loud. Start it out, "Dear Sophie, I've received your letter and I want you to know –"'

She pondered a moment, then began. She was finished several minutes before her allotted ten minutes was up.

'Well, *that* was interesting!' she exclaimed. And she read me Mr Bad Boss's 'letter', which essentially said, 'Hey, this is who I am in the role of boss, and I'm not going to change. You can talk to me all you want to, but it won't do you any good. I'll still behave this way. Here's some good news, though – people tend to get promoted quickly out of my department, and if you stay the course you won't have to deal with me much longer.'

'Come back to your own chair,' I said, 'and write a third letter *to* yourself, *from* your Wise Self. Tell yourself what will be best for you to do next.'

Sophie nodded and began to write. Her Wise Self told her to detach, ignore as much as possible, accurately document her ideas and keep her eyes and ears open for potential opportunities for promotion or transfer.

Four months later, Sophie was transferred, with a promotion in pay and title.

Other journal techniques that particularly lend themselves to identification, clarification and resolution through a Series of Three include:

- **Clustering** – Create a 'mind map' from a central word or phrase. Scan the cluster (also known as a 'mind-map' or 'spidergram'), write a synthesis or integration piece, in which you bring together the different elements of the cluster, and notice where the energy or process seems to be constellated. Bring that word, phrase or concept forward as the central word for a second cluster. Repeat. This gives a visual map of your thought process. For extra visual boost, colour-code the clusters with pencils or transparent markers.

- **Sentence stems** – Complete a sentence, such as 'What I really want or need to do is…', several or many different ways. Asterisk the one response that either seems to attract or repel you the most. In Sophie's case, it was '…detach from the drama'. Take that response and turn it into a second sentence stem: 'To detach from the drama, I could…' Again, choose the one response that pulls you or pushes you away. Sophie's second list included '…document my good ideas'. She then wrote a third sentence stem on 'Ideas I need to document' and ended up with a task list.

- **AlphaPoems** – AlphaPoems are discussed in Chapter 1. Particularly when the entire alphabet, A–Z, is used as the spine of the poem, an AlphaPoem can be an effective Series of Three. Find the line, image or phrase in the poem that feels the most 'juicy' and use it, or a variation, as a title for the next AlphaPoem. In the second poem, there may be a line where the poem seems to turn. Pull that line out and again use it as the starting place for a third poem (see also p.46 for more on AlphaPoems).

- **Five (ten)-minute sprints** – Write fast and furious for five or ten minutes on any topic. Review, and underline or circle words or phrases that seem to jump out. Begin a second timed write with these words, phrases or themes. Repeat the process for a third write. At the end, spend another five or ten minutes reading all three writes and synthesising them. This is an excellent way to generate creative flow for fiction or poems.

'This is a Story of My Birth...'[1]   *Maria Antoniou*

The seed for this exercise was planted in autumn 2001 as I sat in the out-patients department of the Royal Sussex Hospital waiting to have a blood test. I was reading a novel I'd brought to take my mind off the hard plastic chair, the nervous chatter of other patients and the smell of sickness. I don't remember the title of the novel, or who wrote it. I do remember that the book didn't appeal to me, and that I didn't make it past the first few pages. But it was those pages that held value for me. In them, the narrator told the story of his birth. And I instantly wanted to write mine too.

I put down the novel and got out my notebook. I jotted down things I had been told, imagined and perhaps remembered about the day that I was born. I pieced together fragments of 'fact' (the date, the place...) and of 'fiction' (the existence of a twin, the whereabouts of my father...), creating a patchwork story of my birth. But then I was called for my blood test.

Several days later I reread my notes. This time I analysed: whose story is this? Is it my story or the stories of others? Is the story real or imagined? What does this story tell me about my origins and my identity? About my place in society? What does it tell me about my relationships with my mother and my father? How does it differ from past stories I may have told about my birth, or the stories I may tell in the future? Is this story just a product of my current life experience? What are the benefits of writing *my own* birth story, to exist alongside the accounts of others? What are the personal benefits? And the socio-political ones?

I am still answering these questions.

I have developed this exercise so that it can be used by others, either individually, one-to-one, or with groups, to explore the stories of their birth.

How this exercise could be used in a workshop
This exercise could be used with diverse individuals and groups, including new mothers; those wanting to examine family relationships; those wanting to explore their origins and identity; and those feeling 'stuck' in their lives. The exercise may stir strong emotions, so it is advisable that an

---

1   Parts of this piece are adapted from Antoniou, A. (2000) *Writing my body: exploring methods for articulating embodiment.* Doctoral thesis. Manchester: University of Manchester.

experienced facilitator leads the group. I have not suggested a time frame as this will be different for each group.

- Seat participants in a circle, either on chairs or on the floor.

- Go around the circle, with each participant calling out a word they associate with the subject of birth. Continue for three or four rounds of the circle.

- Invite the group to individually write down, in note form, anything they remember, have been told or imagine about either being born or giving birth. Ask them to include where and when the birth took place, the people involved and any sights, smells, tastes, sounds or feelings they associate with the event.

- Next, invite them to shape the notes into a story, beginning with the line 'This is a story of my birth...' or 'This is the story of X's birth...'.

- Invite participants to read out their stories, without discussion.

- When everyone has taken their turn, initiate discussion on their experiences of writing the stories, any associated feelings or memories which came up as they wrote, and the personal and social implications of writing our own birth stories.

This exercise could be extended in several ways, including:

1. a guided visualisation on the experience of being born, immediately followed by stream-of-consciousness writing

2. inviting participants to write a fantasy tale about their birth.

> **This is a story of my birth...** I was born on Saturday 14 October 1972. At 5 a.m. Sun Libra, moon Capricorn, Virgo ascending. Plaistow Maternity Hospital, London. I weighed 6lb $3\frac{1}{2}$oz. My head was too big to fit through my mum's vagina. The doctor sliced her flesh to get me out. And then he stitched her up again. My dad wasn't at my birth. He was on nightshift, a railway porter at Paddington station. I was born two weeks prematurely. I had jaundice at birth, my skin was the colour of weak tea. My parents carried me from the hospital to the house they had bought that summer. They had been married for exactly 11 months on the day of my birth. I was conceived in Scarborough in January 1972. They'd gone to stay with my dad's uncle who

owned a chip shop. It was supposed to be their honeymoon. But my granddad went with them on the trip. I was named Maria after my paternal grandmother, following Cypriot tradition. If I'd been born a boy I'd have been called Antonis. After my dad's dad. I don't have a middle name. I began my life as a twin. He died before he had fingers or a face. I've always known it was a 'he'. Perhaps I remember him? Perhaps I feel his presence – the missing half of me? A medium told my sister we have a brother 'in spirit'. But my mum says I have no twin, she had no miscarriage, it was 'just a bit of bleeding'. I was breast-fed for a week before my mum ran out of milk.

Voices from the Streets: The Brighton Big Issue Writing Group
Dominique De-Light

Daily, I watch passers by who are richer than me,
Going for meals in cafés where I can't afford tea.
There's blokes with women more witty and pretty
Than those girls that stop and chat with me
While all the time I try not to berate
Those better off people, who, to be honest, I hate
People in shopping malls where I can't window shop
Security staring at me: I get in a strop.
They go to expensive restaurants to eat,
Whilst I'm lucky to get a tin of processed meat.
(Martin Curtis)

The word 'homeless' conjures up images of old tramps with cans of strong beer. Few attending the Brighton Big Issue writing group fit into this category, the majority being far more diverse: young, old, women, men, artists, travellers, ex-businessmen, teenagers, those who are well educated and those with no education. All are at the bottom of the social ladder. The only thing they have in common: they've run out of places to turn and feel ignored by society.

Many are ex-prisoners who've lost their accommodation whilst inside; more than half have mental health issues; many have used drugs in the past, many still do. The majority have suffered some form of abuse as children. Most are classified as dual diagnosis – battling with drugs and mental health issues and homelessness all at the same time. They are complex clients with complex needs.

Though students are male and female, aged between 18 and 80, the core members are men between 25 and 45. In the four years I've run the group, between 5 and 15 people attend every week. Roughly half are regulars, but as it is a two-hour drop-in, many come once or twice before they, or their lives, move on. Roughly a third have not written since leaving school, another third's only experience is writing letters and diaries, whilst the remainder have attended writing groups in prison or completed post-compulsory education courses at some level. The group is as diverse in social and educational levels as are their reasons for ending up on the street.

Established for over eight years – but sadly closed down in October 2005 due to lack of funding – the group was inspired by the 'Streetlights' pages – the 'voice of the homeless' – in *The Big Issue* magazine. Members write rants, reviews, poetry and short stories, submitting them weekly for publication. Those that make it into print receive payment.

One regular, who'd never written before, now uses writing as an alternative to self-harming. Another, severely withdrawn and depressed, has been encouraged by his characters' adventures to have adventures of his own: accessing the internet and travelling abroad. One member, believed to have paranoid schizophrenia, was re-diagnosed as exhibiting 'learnt behaviour'. His expression through poetry and regular group attendance was considered a stabilising influence on his condition. As one student wrote:

Anytime Will Do by Martin Edwards

Why should we be afraid of madness?
After all, we've all been mad before,
Few of us have ever found the room.
So much better if we let insanity take us to happier living,
Other worlds seem user friendly,
You never know what's round the bend.
Amongst a forest of stark ravens and march hares,
Larks a people who've lost their marbles,
Who know which plot they live at?

Writing enables self-expression. Publication gains recognition from others. Creativity raises self-esteem and self-respect. This is why they come. Every student emphasises their individuality when dropping in for the first time. All insist they are there simply for professional literary advice. Yet many write purely for release rather than to develop their writing skills.

Employed as a professional writer to facilitate their creative development, my work combines literary critique with informal counselling. Though many come for the therapeutic benefits, it's vital for the group's success that it's not billed as therapeutic or educational, for many of this client group have had negative experiences of both.

Many rebel against structure, so I do not set exercises. They come with ideas or I suggest some. These arise naturally through conversation about their lives, their experiences or their viewpoint. Trust is key. One member, now a regular, hung outside the door for weeks claiming he couldn't write. I talked to him more each time, finally asking him to write 'what he felt'. Since then, he's written pieces regularly and is published roughly every two months. Often, a reluctant member is enticed in with a cup of tea and I just ask 'for a few words in return'. Many, once putting pen to paper, don't stop, words flowing like a river through a burst dam. More confident members chose to share their work with the group but most are reluctant. They show me, wanting feedback, but prefer others only to see their efforts if they are printed. Many are surprised and touched by the recognition publication gains them from their peers.

To an outsider the group may appear chaotic: no exercises, no set students, no formal group sharing of work – difficult with changing members and people paranoid from years of drug use or poor mental health. Yet there are clear parameters. First and foremost, everyone is accepted whatever their past. How they came to be there is not important; their writing is the focus. To ensure everyone feels safe and welcome, clear boundaries are established. Everyone must be treated with respect. Intense discussions may occur but they must never get confrontational. A calm, holding environment is key. Many have had problems with boundaries in the past, so group rules are restated clearly and often, in a friendly fashion.

Equally important, with changing members, is the stability I provide. I start and end the group in a similar way; I greet people with the offer of a drink, the pens and paper are always in the same place. Time and time again, they tell me, they're sick of being seen as cases and want to be treated as individuals. Absolutely crucial is ensuring everyone gets one-to-one time, that critiques are tailored to the individual and assumptions are not made.

This is a group for people to be heard: if they feel they've been missed out, attention-grabbing antics occur. These are to be avoided at all costs; though usually manageable, they can be potentially dangerous. As the facilitator, I have to be professional whilst not appearing too authoritative, caring but not personally involved, encouraging but honest. Members with little respect for authority, structure or rules will soon kick up a fuss if they feel you are 'faking it'. This client group is used to being brushed aside, placated or ignored. Everyone needs to be acknowledged. We write for we feel we have something to say. All of us, whatever our situation, client, professional or academic, need an audience. We need to be heard. Our job is to ensure society listens.

Configurations of Self   *Jeannie Wright*

It was six o'clock. At the end of a long training day, some students and their tutor sat in a circle to work on 'personal development'. The timetabling and venue, a damp portakabin near the car park, were not of their choosing. Outside it was already dark and inside the overhead strip lighting created a greenish, aquarium-like gloom. It was November. The students were mostly female. They were, for the most part, the first generation of their families to come into higher education. The tutor looked around at drained faces and wished she could send them all home, or better on holiday to somewhere warmer. She took a deep breath.

'We're going to work on our own on these sheets of paper first of all,' she said.

After weeks of wrangling she had persuaded 'the office' to buy large sheets of pink, purple, blue, green and yellow paper. There were some groans and mumblings but, as usual, the tutor joined in and took a sheet of yellow paper and some felt tips. She drew a line across it, wavy and purple, and then started to write. The instructions for their work together were on an overhead, and began as follows:

> Draw a line across the page and write the names of three people who know you well on this line. The names could be those of family and friends but might not be – it's your choice.

> Pause for a moment and think about how you would describe yourself. Then write what these people would say about you if asked to describe you.

The tutor wrote:

> How would I describe myself?
>
> *Disappointed idealist.*
>
> How would others who know me well describe me?
>
> *Considerate, compliant, calm – all the 'c's? – creative?*

She had jumped ahead of the instructions which continued:

> Above the line write/draw against each name the positives; for example: 'she's considerate and always thinks of others'.
>
> Below the line, write/draw what they might want to change in you; for example: 'she's never stood up for herself enough'.
>
> Finally, reflecting on these qualities of yourself, what would you like to change?

Looking around, the tutor saw that the entire group, 24 of them this evening, was now engaged with the writing and drawing. She went back to her own sheet of paper:

> What would I like to change?
>
> *The grind – putting up with the unacceptable.*
>
> *I am wasting whole years of my life on public sector, portakabin grime and administrative absurdities. Institutional procedures keep me tired and I'm getting old.*

The vehemence of the words shocked her. She had used a thick orange pen and the writing was large and as if stamped on the paper. She blinked and looked at her watch.

'We've got another half an hour,' she said. 'Could you join up with a partner or small group of people you want to reflect on your writing and drawing with?'

A few people were still writing, but the energy now in the room could be seen and heard. Not for the first time the tutor wished she could join in – participate in rather than facilitate one of the small groups. She'd have to wait.

Context – Personal/professional development in any appropriate course of training; for example: social work, counselling and psychotherapy, or any kind of people work. I have also suggested this exercise for clients who use writing therapy, or as a way of starting work on 'self' with face-to-face counselling clients. Although the title is drawn from person-centred theory (based on the work of Carl Rogers), it fits with most orientations with an interest in self-awareness as part of the therapeutic relationship. If time runs out, the reflective writing can always be suggested as 'homework'...

Timing – From two hours (minimum) to half a day.

Lindy's Story   *Kate Evans*

'It feels good to get some of the anger out on paper,' says Lindy. 'Instead of having it swirling around inside me.' And it is obvious from the slight relaxation of her posture that some of her intense rage has been released.

Last term Lindy was one of the five regulars at the creative writing group I facilitate at Scarborough Survivors, but at the start of this term I was told that she was back in hospital. Our group, funded by the Workers Education Association, had been meeting each Wednesday for almost a year and I missed Lindy's questioning, her compassion for the other members of the group (including me) and the incisive honesty of her writing. I hoped her stay in hospital would not last too long, though the news I had of her was not encouraging.

It is break time on the fourth week of term and we have gone, as we always do, down to the Scarborough Survivors' coffee bar. Lindy walks in. She has come straight from the hospital. I can feel her tension and anxiety like it's whipping up the air around us. She sits by one of the Scarborough Survivor members she knows and explains her distress. The psychiatrist discharged her without consulting her, saying that she would get better support with the crisis team. But she doesn't trust them as they drew up a care plan without even meeting her.

It looks like she will go round and round with her confusion and frustration. I suggest she joins us for the second half of the creative writing. She says she might as well.

We start off with some music and three minutes of sprint writing to bring people back to a creative state of mind. I then recap on Roger McGough's 'The Map' (McGough 1999) and Sharon Olds' 'On the Subway' (Olds 1987), the narrative poems we looked at earlier. I suggest people pick a line that they like from one of the poems and write their own story for today.

Lindy cries during the music and says she can't listen to it or write anything. When I ask her what her words might be at this point, she says 'lonely' and 'isolated'.

When we return to the narrative poems, everyone except Lindy starts writing quickly. She rereads the poems and she stares at her paper. After some minutes I am about to go and talk to her when she starts to write. Once begun it doesn't seem like she will stop even when the others begin to share their work.

The last to go, Lindy reads 'Trust Me, Trust Me Not' which expresses graphically her frustration and anger at not being able to express her opinion to her psychiatrist and not being able to stop her discharge from hospital.

The others react well to it; one says that being sent home is always a difficult time and that she has a file full of poetry that she wrote at hers.

I ask Lindy how she feels and she says it's better to have the anger out in front of her, which can be seen in her body language. I also suggest I keep 'Trust Me, Trust Me Not' for her (as I am afraid she might destroy it) and she lets me take it.

The following week, Lindy is there again, in a much calmer mood. She says that the previous session helped her and that she is pleased I preserved 'Trust Me, Trust Me Not' for her, as she would have screwed it up and now she wants to work on it. She has written a further poem characterising her psychiatrist as a ventriloquist's dummy which causes much hilarity and encourages the others to talk about their relationships with their psychiatrists. Lindy comments, 'It's therapeutic to laugh at your psychiatrist sometimes.'

Even at her lowest ebb, Lindy was able to confirm something very important about what we were all doing together. Rose Flint describes the therapeutic relationship as a 'fragile space' (Flint 2000). In my way of working I aim to create a space for exploration which is both safe and surely very fragile indeed as it is difficult to predict what my travelling companions will bring with them and where this exploration will take us. I do not consider it my job to direct this so much as to accompany and to offer choices along the way. People will often write what they have to write whatever the exercise or session I have planned. I remain open to and want to encourage that. I don't want to suggest that there is no preparation or purposefulness in my approach; certainly there are effects or issues that I would like to elicit, though I also want to be receptive to all others.

As with anyone setting out on a complex journey, however, I feel it is my responsibility to be as prepared as I possibly can be. I have strategies (discussed beforehand with participants) for if crises should arise, and I am committed to continually developing my own skills and to seeking the advice, support and supervision that I need.

I would like to think that coming into the relaxed supportive atmosphere of the group and doing the two exercises I proposed did help Lindy to deal more effectively with her anger. It is difficult to be certain. What was observable, however, was that the activity of writing down her experiences in poetic form had an immediately calming effect whereas talking about it to a trusted acquaintance downstairs in the coffee bar did not.

Music followed by three minutes' sprint writing
This is an exercise that I use frequently to get people 'limbered up' and relaxed, to make a break between the real world and the writing world. I try and use music which either has no words or has words in another language. This usually ensures that it is not known by the students, so will be free of immediate associations, and that there are no recognisable words to influence what the student writes. My favourite for a first meeting is 'First Cry' by the Native American singer Sharon Birch. Usually I will try and choose music which matches the theme or feel of the workshop: a wistful piece to create an atmosphere of reflection, a more upbeat one to encourage activity. I'm not entirely sure if this is an exercise of my own making. It was certainly inspired by the need to encourage the use of all senses in writing and teaching. As well as the idea that listening to music excites the right-hand – our more imaginative, intuitive – side of the brain.

Trust Me, Trust Me Not *by Lindy Herrington*

By the time I enter the room I feel small and frightened
I deliberately sit where he can't stare through me as before
Then he confronts me, first with words, then with silence
Our words clash as I try to say how I feel
The others start to speak
But once again he raises his voice
and dilutes our voices to nothingness.
For the last time I hear him say he's decided
I've decided to discharge you today
You'll get more help at home than in here
I guarantee it.

I disagree but the words won't leave my mouth.

Trust me. Trust me not.

Face of a China Doll (unfinished) by Lindy Herrington

His master lifts him carefully
from the small suitcase that is his home
and kits him out in the Ladybird range from Woolworths
Suit and tie, nicely polished shoes – size 4

He has the face of a china doll
pale – almost white, and the handshake of a wet fish
Now he's ready to start work
See how you get on without me, his master says

From a distance he looks real
He comes to the waiting room for his next patient
but no one comes

He doesn't know that his master forgot to connect his eyes

He almost gets away with it as the new psychiatrist.

One-to-One Creative Writing Session: Writing Emerging from Personal Spoken Experience   *Fiona Hamilton*

In one-to-one creative writing sessions when I have been able to establish a rapport with the participant over several sessions, I like to try to allow the writing to emerge from what is spoken or felt in the moment.

For this to happen, I have to trust more and plan less. Trust that I can listen carefully and respond precisely and authentically, allow space for whatever artistic material begins to form in words, and be willing to draw on my own creative senses to help the participant engage with and shape their material.

Here I will describe some of the process that occurred in working with a woman called Maeve (the name and details have been changed to preserve anonymity) in the hospital where she was receiving treatment for cancer. This was a project offering free creative writing sessions to patients, carers and staff, funded by Writing in Healthcare, an organisation based in

Bristol, and supported by Arts Council England and Awards for All. We had use of a small, windowless room, containing two chairs and a telephone (which I unplugged). I brought clipboards to lean on, paper and pens.

Maeve had written many poems over the years 'but done nothing with them'. Now that she was off work, she felt this could be an opportunity to develop her writing.

Maeve liked to talk for a while at the beginning of each session, about how her week had been, or how she was feeling. On this occasion Maeve told me that she felt tired. The day before she had been to visit a friend in Cardiff. She had felt very excited on the train on the way there. This was the first time she had been to visit her old friend since her diagnosis. On the way home, however, she had felt irritable and tired. At night she dreamed about getting on a train with a lot of heavy luggage and feeling worried that she wouldn't be able to get her suitcases off the train at the right stop. Then she saw the luggage roll out of the train and into a field.

In a previous session, Maeve had described a holiday in Northumberland, where she had collected stones from the beach. One of the stones had become precious to her – she found holding its cold smooth surface reassuring during the discomforts of chemotherapy.

While she was talking, I listened attentively. I was allowing Maeve's description of her experience to sink in and noting the effect on me. I had very visual impressions of what she was telling me, and a phrase came into my mind – 'This journey begins'.

I turned the phrase over in my thoughts while continuing to listen. I decided to use it as a starting point for writing. I invited Maeve to write it down and build a piece around it, repeating it a few times. I gave ten minutes for writing.

This is what she wrote:

> This journey begins
> One day fourteen hundred years ago
> In a street
> In a house
> In a room
>
> This journey begins
> With one of my ancestors
> Opening one eye
> Then the other

> On a day of sunshine, shouts, running,
> Soup, dogs, conversations,
> A joke, a cut finger, a kiss
>
> This journey begins
> With somebody
> Getting out of bed
> Tipping a small ball over the edge of a staircase
> And letting it clunk down each step

When I asked her how it had been to write this way, she said that the words 'just seemed to come out'. She commented that she 'didn't know where they came from'. She laughed, and then added, looking at what she had written, 'And I don't know where I came from.'

She said that she had recently been thinking about members of her own family – her parents, aunts and uncles – and she supposed that her writing was about making sense of where she came from, and how she related to past generations.

I asked her if she would like to develop the writing further. She replied that she wanted to 'get away' from her familiar writing voice, and try some alternative styles, perhaps lighter or even frivolous in tone.

We talked about experimenting with a child's voice, and inventing words playfully. We looked at the list in her piece:

> sunshine, shouts, running,
> soup, dogs, conversations,
> a joke, a cut finger, a kiss

and talked about taking one of these that suggested an incident from childhood which she would like to write about. She chose 'soup' and I suggested that if she wanted to she might jot down some child's-eye observations of the incident to bring to the next session.

To the next session a week later Maeve brought a five-line poem made up of invented words, rhythmic and playful, in the voice of a child who is eagerly tasting tomato soup her granny has made her, and spilling it on her clothes.

In later sessions, she returned to consider the darker feelings and fears expressed through her dream, but for now she was pleased to have found a way of expressing her more playful and childlike side, whilst continuing to explore her family relationships and history.

CHAPTER 7

Different Masks

Edited by Victoria Field

Jung was the first to use the Greek word for an actor's mask – 'persona' – to refer to the different parts we play in our social worlds. Most of us are conscious of the varied roles we play in the world and the expectations of others that go with many of these roles. Society could not function without the shared understanding of what it means to be, for example, a teacher, a bus driver, a doctor or a student. Most of the time, our feelings and behaviour are not in conflict with the roles we are asked to play nor with our inner selves. At other times, however, the discrepancy can be acutely felt and there can be an urgent need to find the 'real me'.

Arguably, one of the goals of therapy and therapeutic writing is to encourage better integration of the different personae – or masks – that all of us wear during daily life. People talk about wanting to find 'themselves' or say that certain roles they are required to play are 'not really me'. The challenge is to be able to embrace and celebrate our complex and multiple selves whilst still feeling authentic, integrated and real. The popularity of books and courses that focus on self-discovery are testimony to the commonly held idea that there is an essential self that is there to be uncovered. Therapeutic writing can be useful in reflecting aspects of ourselves back to ourselves, and the results are often surprising and illuminating.

In a therapeutic writing setting, even the initial acknowledgement of multiple selves can be freeing. Society, including those closest to us, colludes in the myth of consistency, both within ourselves and over time. Most people have experienced, say, a mother who refuses to acknowledge that her adult offspring may no longer like baked beans or a husband who is horrified at the thought of his wife cutting her hair or gaining or losing weight. One way into the idea of a hidden self is to invite participants to say one thing that is true about themselves and one thing that is untrue. This is a good ice-breaker to do orally at the beginning of a session and one that I often use with children. They are thrilled at actually being invited to tell a lie and the exercise immediately takes them into creating fantasies about themselves. Graham Hartill explores this further below in I am True, I am False, I am Impossible.

Another way of exploring this multiplicity of selves is to engage with the opposites within our personalities. If we are female, then how does our male side, the animus, think, feel and behave? If we are 'good boys', what is it that our bad boy would like to do? Clearly, many elements of our personalities fall along a continuum rather than existing as a pair of polar opposites. Nevertheless, the use of these opposites can sometimes jolt participants into a new way of looking at themselves. Alison Clayburn offers an exercise in creating a character who is the opposite of the writer in Character Creation from Self and Opposite.

In our society which prioritises the rational, there is often a perceived conflict between our emotional and spontaneous sides and the intellectual and considered side. Alison Clayburn explores this in her exercise Head and Heart. As well as the satisfaction of creating poems, the results of this could be used for participants to reflect on the balance of head and heart influence in their own lives.

Inevitably, there are parts of ourselves with which we engage most readily and other parts that are denied or rejected. Freud theorised that those unexpressed and, possibly, unconscious areas of our personality may lead us to repeat unwelcome patterns of behaviour. Bringing these areas into consciousness may illuminate unacknowledged motivations and give the possibility of change. Jung developed the idea of us having a 'shadow side' to our personality, with all its connotations of mystery and darkness, and this is one that Reinekke Lengelle explores in Writing the Shadow. She finds that, by engaging closely with the shadow or unacceptable side of our personalities, we can often find insights into how they can, in fact, help and support us. Her workshop description applies to a writing group in which the participants seem at ease with themselves – this is an approach that should be handled extremely carefully and only used in a group where an experienced facilitator knows the participants well.

Geri Giebel Chavis presents Two Colour Vignettes which elegantly show how a simple metaphor can reveal aspects of the self which may be obscured by other more noticeable or habitual ways of perceiving ourselves or others. Like many of the pieces in this chapter, hers is concerned with

giving voice to the repressed or not-fully-heard voices within us. Monica
Suswin's account, Contours of the Self, brings in the Gestalt – a way of
engaging with the whole self in the present moment through identification
with an outside object. Objects, like metaphor, can be potent catalysts for
insights into the self and tap in directly to important issues. One of
Monica's group leaves early as a result of realising that she, like the garden
bench she identifies with, does not want to be 'sat on'. The use of objects in
therapeutic writing is explored further in Chapter 3.

   A common finding is that our writing self can often be at odds with the
personae of our everyday self. Writing, especially 'for the drawer', can be
perceived as a transgressive or selfish act by the writer and those around
them. Poet David Hart (personal communication) has asked who this
writing self is and how it relates to our other selves:

> And another group of questions ask who we are. Who are the
> selves who 'experience'? Who are the selves that speak? That
> write? Speaking for myself I am son, brother, parent, writer,
> divorcé, friend, workshop leader, lone walker; in my life there is
> also Anglican priest, theatre critic, arts administrator... I am
> indebted here to Miller Mair's insight that we are each of us a
> 'community of selves'. So, then...which self of us (or various of
> us at different times) makes the poems? Which self is it that
> writes with optimism? Which self puts it aside as of no worth? Is
> it the same self who experiences and who writes, or is there a
> costume drama going on here? If I go for a walk and think to
> write, when I come back and write, is it the same self who writes,
> or does another self take over to do it? Does another self edit it?

The final two workshops described here both encourage participants to
engage with their writer selves. Claire Williamson directly invokes the idea
of a 'writer mask', not just as a persona but as a literal mask that might be
drawn or decorated. She suggests becoming the writer's friend. River
Wolton explores the voice of our inner critic – the one that might appear to
sabotage our attempts at writing. Rather than simply trying to destroy the
critic, she looks at ways its energy can be harnessed in passionate tango.

   The dance is an apt metaphor for our relationship with our many selves
and the challenge is how to choreograph their different styles and impulses
into a lively, challenging but ultimately harmonious ensemble.

I am True, I am False, I am Impossible   *Graham Hartill*

I once had a conversation with Prince Charles about pig farming. I used to be a bit of an expert on the subject and, as he was getting into organic pig-breeding on one of his estates, he naturally wanted to know more. I was the one to talk to so he asked to meet me. He took me to one side and asked me all sorts of questions; I answered him as best I could and afterwards, of course, the press wanted to know everything that had passed between us. Well, I didn't tell them much as I reckoned it was just between me and Charles. He thanked me enthusiastically for all the help I had given him and told me it would help him a great deal in his work.

Actually that's not what happened. To be honest I did something a bit naughty to Prince Charles once. I was working in this hospice for a summer job when I was a student and he came to visit. There was a whole entourage with him of course; it was a whirlwind visit to Cirencester. As he was going around pressing the flesh and chatting to everyone he was offered a cup of tea and a piece of cake. What he didn't know was that I had baked a hash cookie especially for him which he duly accepted. He ate it with relish and carried on with his duties in his usual amicable way; in fact he seemed even more friendly after that and seemed to really enjoy listening to all the old wives' tales he was getting told. Then he flew off in his helicopter and it was a nice sunny day so I hope he enjoyed the view as he spun away over the river and the meadows and the motorway flyover.

That's not true either.

Maybe.

This exercise can be an effective and very funny ice-breaker for any new group. Everyone has to write down two or three paragraphs about themselves, one or more of which must be true, one or more of which must be false. The other members have to guess, through open discussion, which is which. The game for each writer is to fool the rest by writing about something which seems 'out-of-character' but which is actually true. This will usually be met with gasps of surprise, laughter and lots of questions when revealed. The false stories on the other hand must be written credibly.

The game can be a harmless way to learn about each other's lives and personalities while opening up some issues to do with writing fact and fiction. Projections and presumptions can be aired through humour and ideas for more developed pieces can be released. Issues about the imagination can also be discussed: why did someone try to pretend they actually carried out that particular fantasy? What kind of self were they imagining there? How good were they at fooling us? And what was it about the way they wrote it that convinced us, or not?

Go deeper. You could go back to this exercise in future sessions. Expand on the issues and revelations raised initially, both in terms of content and writing skills. Think about who we are, or think we are, really and how we perceive each other, and ourselves. What roles and personae do we tend to assume in our lives? What fantasies are waiting to be fulfilled? Are our memories reliable? What's possible? And what is not?

Are we the facts of our lives? Or more the imagination in which we live them?

Character Creation from Self and Opposite
Alison Clayburn

> Angus is a tall thin vegan who enjoys running up hills and has a fondness for snails – as wildlife, not eating them of course. I met him in the 1990s at a Buddhist retreat centre in the Scottish hills. I was on a group writing retreat – but he wasn't part of our group, and wasn't at all keen to join in because he's not at all creative – in fact I'm not sure he knows what the word means. I found him amusing – but a bit boring; not surprising as he's very different from me, my opposite in fact. When we first talked about each other (privately) we were mutually critical – I found myself defending my well-endowed physique, my dietary habits and my lack of enthusiasm for even climbing the hills, let alone running up them. But then we had a proper conversation, by the end of which he had persuaded me that a little adjustment to my diet and some kind of regular exercise, especially in that lovely Scottish air, was not a bad idea, and I had managed to formulate very clear ideas on why creative activity, especially writing, was important to me and others in the writing group. I might even have persuaded him to have a go himself – but I'll never know, because he's just a figment of my imagination.

Divide your page into two columns. In the left-hand column write a list of ten words or phrases to describe yourself. Be factual as well as subjective and focus on the present moment. For example, 'Right now I am female, fat, creative and tired, but I hope the last one changes!'

Then write an opposite list in the right-hand column. You can describe the opposites as you see them – although male/female are a bit rigid! My opposites would be male, thin, devoid of ideas and full of energy.

These are the initial directions for a workshop I developed from a group experiment. It can be done all in one session, or with later steps for homework if it's part of an ongoing course.

Then give your opposite a name and write a free-flow monologue from his/her point of view. Focus on your present situation, as if you were both in the same space. Very interesting if it's a writing workshop! Let him/her express his/her thoughts in general and then include what he/she thinks of you.

Write a response. How do you feel about him/her? Give yourself equal time and space.

Write an interactive scene, bringing out the relationship between you and your opposite. Give yourself another name and refer to yourself in the third person.

It can help to ask reflective questions afterwards and these are my suggestions, the first of which can aid the development of writing skills alongside the self-exploration:

- How well do you feel the different characters were portrayed in the scene?

- What did you learn about yourself from this interaction?

- What did you learn from the whole exercise?

Here's an example of the kind of writing that can emerge:

> In the early 2000s, in London, Clint met Mavis... As a tall, slim man in good health who described himself as laid back, curious, persistent-stubborn, cooperative, friendly and philosophical, he was very unlike Mavis – who was small and fat, in bad health, uptight and, Clint felt, lacked involvement in the world. He saw her as someone who would give up easily on projects, was unfriendly and unwilling to assist others, but he also knew she had trouble making sense of the world... As they shared a bag of chips on the way to a music festival in Kew Gardens, they talked...

> 'Mave, I think you could handle failure; mistakes and failure help us grow...if we learn from them.' Clint strained. 'I don't want the rest of these chips.'

> 'Good, I'll 'ave 'em!' exclaimed Mavis lustfully.

> 'Mavis, you're getting fatter.'

'Oh, shut yer face, you're far from perfect, I bet you never tell anyone that you love them.'

Somewhat stunned, Clint stammered, 'Jesus, you're right…how did you know?'

Head and Heart   *Alison Clayburn*

It is summer 2004, the ninth session in my 12-week course in creative writing for self-discovery at Mary Ward Centre. This course attracts a wide variety of individuals. For some, personal development is paramount; for others, improving their writing is more important. I enjoy the challenge of these dual goals, which are made clear at the start of the course.

Now it's the time to get stuck in to one of my favourites – Head and Heart. I've used it in other courses and in one-off workshops with Survivors Poetry. The idea originated in my year of intensive psycho-synthesis training about ten years ago, but of course I've fiddled with it. Psychosynthesis is a useful technique in bringing the different elements of the personality into harmony.

I introduce the exercise. This is a really familiar 'split' and it enables the students to further the use of imagery and dialogue we've already practised. I tell them I am going to give them prompts, asking them to write first about head and then about heart. I find oral prompts effective in producing quick and spontaneous raw material – an advantage of being in a class or workshop rather than working from written directions. I ask them to write one short phrase for each response. The prompts are:

> What does my head sound like?
> What does my head smell like?
> What does my head look like?
> What does my head feel (tactile) like?

Then:

> What is it doing?

And then I repeat the prompts for 'my heart'.

We share some responses in the whole group. As time is limited, I just ask them to share the *smell* and *doing* images, as these are likely to be the most idiosyncratic and interesting for a hasty hearing. There is time to do the next part of the activity in class, which is to select the most striking images, consolidate the descriptions of head and heart and to both read out and discuss them with two others in a small group.

The next part of the activity is to set up a dialogue between head and heart and see what they have to say to each other, what their relationship is like.

I ask them to do this for homework and then to write a poem – I suggest that they write one stanza on head, one on heart, and then a stanza bringing them together.

The following week we share results in class, as well as reflecting on process and discussing it. These are some of the poems that were written, with a quick thumbnail sketch of the writers:

> My head looks like an aerial map of Milton Keynes South
> 1st Avenue, 2nd Avenue, 3rd Avenue, blah! blah! blah!
> trudging along towards terminal boredom like a yeti and a robot's only son
> who's chosen a career in the Civil Service as it's marginally better than dying.
>
> My heart tastes like the juices of the artichokes from the deli on Cold Bath Road
> pumping out love like a newborn child, it's the ache in Jane Kerr's panda eyes
> it's the overwhelming silence in a field of praying Buddhists scampering around corners on its way to God knows where.
>
> My head and my heart, me and my brother,
> Lennon and McCartney, Simon and Garfunkel,
> a melting pot of love and hate like all the great partnerships are
> a bickering old couple who have finally called a truce.

That poem was written by A, a man in his thirties. He has done a lot of creative work – art, music and writing – as part of his process of recovery from addiction. He writes freely, self-defines as a creative child, finds being in a group enlightening and supportive.

Head and Heart

Sensible, smooth, cold,
Rigid, odourless
Tasteless, featureless
Silent grey steel ball.

Fun, shaped, fun-shaped,
Wobbly, sweet smell,
Strawberry flavoured
Food treat of childhood.

Both are part of me;
Sense, fun co-exist.
Lose one, lose myself,
My humanity.

That poem was written by M, who is in his twenties. He is an editor who wants to rediscover creative writing – he came to the course for a push to create spontaneously.

For other settings I might use this poem of mine first to give more imaging practice – again with oral prompts. It came from an exercise in writing a metaphor for a feeling or state of mind, the prompts being:

What does it smell like?
What does it sound like?
Where does it live?
What is it doing?

This Black Cloud Has a Life of Its Own *by Alison Clayburn*

It smells like a mattress, left outside
for five days in a garbage strewn alley,
then moved to an overheated room
where cats have been pissing in a corner.

It sounds like a high-pitched squeal of metal
relentlessly grating on other metal,
scouring grooves which are going to fill up
with horse manure and then inedible fungi.

It lives about three inches down a gutter
in a narrow street in Leytonstone, which
has a dead tree overhanging it and
a one-eyed dog shitting in it every day.

It rubs itself against a rusty drainpipe,
trying to imitate the orgasm it had
five years ago when it was, for almost
two weeks, in a good relationship. (Clayburn 2002)

Writing the Shadow: An Exercise for Exorcising the Demons Within
Reinekke Lengelle

My father used to say: 'Within ardent denial, hides a confession.' I'm reminded of this whenever I catch myself saying: 'I'm not *that*. I may be this, but for heaven's sake, not *that*!'

The collection of selves we disown was described by Carl Jung as the archetypal shadow. These sub-selves can be likened to actors who are playing out the more undesirable parts in the theatre of our lives. And yet these unwanted sub-personalities may come bearing gifts if we are willing to delve into the muck a little and see them integrated into our greater being.

Inspired by Jung's exploration of the shadow, American self-help author Debbie Ford (1998) has paid particular attention to the phenomenon of disowned selves and developed insights into how we put into practice the idea of 'owning' our 'whole story'. I've developed a one-page writing exercise that brings some of these insights together.

There are about 12 students in my 'Writing for the Heart' class. It's late autumn and we've already had a decent snowfall. From the classroom window we can see the evergreens loaded with the white stuff and the sun is fading fast. This is the third Wednesday night of the course and I've prepared the material to work on the shadow with them tonight. It's never a topic I introduce on the first or second night, but eventually a sense of inner timing tells me they're ready to try it and I'm ready to share it.

I start by asking my students to choose someone in the class to work with and instruct them to take turns writing down all the positive or admirable traits they could see in the other. It doesn't matter if the partners haven't worked together before or have barely met: 'If you don't feel you know this person well enough, fictionalise,' I tell them.

'Why do we do this exercise?' I ask them. 'The first reason is because it feels good and as writers we can consider giving the gift of words to one another.'

Another reason we try this exercise is because writers must learn to assume things about people: it gives us the ability to create story and fictionalise even if we're initially working with real people.

'The third reason we do this has to do with the principle of projection.' I go on to explain that the list they've made may say just as much (if not more) about themselves or what they aspire to be as it does about the person they've just written about. They laugh a bit sheepishly and look back at the page to verify what I've suggested for themselves. Now, I know they are ready to make the leap into the dark.

'So if what we admire and see in others in the positive is a projection, this may also apply to the nasty stuff. What I'm proposing is that the traits we so despise in others may say a lot about areas in our lives we need to work on.' Some of them laugh pleasantly at being had.

I explain that when we are projecting, there is often a certain emotional charge attached to our finger-pointing ('Remember,' I add jokingly, 'that while you're pointing at someone else, your three remaining fingers are directed back at you'). Next, I ask students to come up with a list of traits they don't like about themselves. Some start writing furiously, while others find it harder to start this way. To help the latter group, I read them a list of Debbie Ford's 'insults' (1998, p.69). It goes something like this: bitch, wimp, lush, jerk, incompetent, unreliable, chaotic, out-of-control, emotional, anal retentive. I suggest that when uncovering a shadow trait, you may find:

- You react strongly to something someone has said to you or about you. What is the label you're reacting to? What would you *not* like said about you? Which label has hurt you in the past? What has made you feel insulted or criticised or rejected?

- You go into strong denial about something and find yourself saying, 'I'm not...' (fill in the blank).

- You label someone else adamantly: for example, 'He's so judgemental.'

A student named Valerie pipes up and says right away: 'I just hate it when I'm called a wimp.' (See her responses to the entire exercise below.) She is an avid mountaineer and, even in the writing she has shared with us previously, she has displayed anything but wimpy behaviour; yet this label plagues her.

I ask each of them to write down the 'offending' label as specifically as possible: 'wimp' (in Valerie's case).

Then we individually explore two or three of the 'worst' labels in greater detail. The instructions for that part of the exercise look something like this: Demystify the label by writing about what it means to you. Being 'a wimp' might mean feeble, ineffective. Explore when you have heard the label before, why you so dislike this word being used in a way that relates to you. What did 'a wimp' mean in your family of origin? Sometimes the initial label one comes up with is only the surface…for instance 'wimp' might be more about being 'unlovable or incompetent'. It is important to identify the label that gives the highest emotional charge.

> In my family I was the youngest and considered the runt. My siblings used to dare me to do things they could already do. If I was too scared or too small to actually do what they said, I'd be called 'a wimp'. I hated that, I hate it to this day. (Valerie)

Explore, even in a very small way, where this label applies to you.

> I do a lot of hiking and have travelled around the world. I'm not a wimp, that's for sure! But one thing that I can say that I'm remotely wimpy about is swimming in cold water. When I go hiking and my friends jump in an ice-cold mountain stream, I don't; I simply wimp out. (Valerie)

Ask how this label is or has served you in some way.

> My friends went down to take a swim near a waterfall in the Rockies. They met up with a grizzly bear… Fortunately no one was hurt or attacked, but I was so grateful that I had not gone with them. So in a small way being a 'wimp' served me. (Valerie)

Later on that evening, her hand goes up again.

> I realise now that being accused of being a wimp as made me over-compensate in life. I have purposely travelled to places that are not considered safe for 'tourists' and have done things that take real courage. I see how not wanting to be called 'a wimp' has given me courage to open new doors. That I believe is a gift too. (Valerie)

Give that part of you a name and describe him or her in more detail. Allow the writing about her to tell you more: don't premeditate. Fictionalise…

> Wimpy Wanda. She owns a scuba suit just to stay out of any cold water. The diving suit even floats. Wanda always double locks her hotel room door. Wimpy Wanda has gone on her hunches whenever she's travelled…she has never broken a bone or been in any major danger while travelling. She…reads the fine print on all contracts and documents. (Valerie)

Finally, I encourage them to write a statement on a piece of paper (one which they could for instance keep in a wallet as a reminder if the topic is particularly timely and pertinent) that says who this inner character is and what sort of gift it brings.

> Wimpy Wanda is a great travelling companion. She keeps me safe. (Valerie)

By the end of the evening, the room feels remarkably relaxed. I invite them to look out for people who irritate and offend them in the upcoming week with the idea of the shadow and projection in mind. For myself, the adage that we are mirrors for one another once again feels more like the truth and less like a philosophical notion. There are rewards to loving all you are and acknowledging your responsibility in the interactions you have; it's one of the messages that comes out of this evening's class.

Sometimes students find it difficult to pinpoint why a label stings or how it applies. I had a young priest in this writing course also. He was a very busy man and over-committed to work obligations. He simply seemed run off his feet. The label that most bothered him was 'incompetent'. He was a well-loved and respected priest and yet this label made him very uncomfortable. He didn't get a chance to explore this in great detail because he had to leave the class early and rush off to another appointment. Perhaps his incompetence lay in simply being unable to say 'no' and schedule his time more realistically.

We can nearly always find a way in which a negative label serves us, even in a minor way. The learning that can be gained is often a relief. 'Bitchy' may really be about 'expressing our truth without fear of reproach'. 'Stupid' might make us realise we're allowed to be imperfect despite the standards we've been holding ourselves to.

Interestingly, once we embrace a 'nasty' piece, its negative influence in our lives often begins to dissipate and the gift attached becomes more apparent. In my student's case this might mean that feeling like a 'wimp' will soon feel more like: 'I am courageous and have good instincts for travelling safely.' And if she wants to 'wimp out', she can do so without the familiar guilt.

And if the Japanese proverb, 'Nothing is as visible as what we try to hide', is true, then pointing the light at ourselves and thereby discovering the shadow may be an even more worthwhile quest.

Two Colour Vignettes   *Geri Giebel Chavis*

Several years ago, I co-facilitated an open-ended psychotherapy group that had been meeting for a number of years at a private psychotherapy clinic in Minneapolis, Minnesota, in the United States. The group, meeting weekly for a 90-minute session, consisted of six to eight adult women and men between the ages of 30 and 50 years. During one particular session, I invited participants to identify a colour that described their present life or state of being. I encouraged them to select the first colour that came to mind as fitting and to free write about the objects, emotions, images or experiences associated with their chosen colour. As an afterthought, I added that they should feel free to opt for a set of two colours if this choice seemed more appropriate. After ten minutes of writing, I invited everyone to share their colour choices and any part of their writings they would be willing to read or discuss.

The particular response that remains distinct in my memory to this day represented a breakthrough for one particular 42-year-old widow who had been struggling with grief and loneliness for the past two years since her husband's death. What was striking is that her immediate first colour choice was 'blue', a reflection of the predominant melancholy feeling state she had repeatedly articulated within the group week after week. But when I added the option of a second colour, she surprised herself and other group members with the choice of 'yellow', proceeding to describe sunlight in her rooms, mellow-coloured flowers and spurts of unanticipated joy. For the first time, she was able to express feelings of peace and even happiness that were dawning within her, feelings she had been reluctant to admit even to herself, because of guilt and because of the grieving mindset she had held for so long. With her colour poem as the catalyst, she could now elaborate on the bright spots in her life that were beginning to move her beyond depression.

A second and completely unrelated colour writing activity took place a few years ago in my private practice with a family of four in an hour-long session. I had been counselling the husband and wife for a period of about three months when I invited them to bring in their two daughters, both teenagers who were clearly aligned with their mother against the father. All four family members were ill at ease in our first family therapy session, until I introduced a simple writing activity involving colour choice. Although none of them had any previous creative writing experiences, they were willing to write when I asked all four family members to select a colour that captures who they are and to free write for a few minutes on anything associated with that colour.

Interestingly enough, despite the alignments that were heightening tension in the marriage and isolating the father from the rest of the family, the father's colour choice of 'dark brown' was closest to the 'black' of the oldest daughter, the one whose conflicts with the father were the most pronounced. The 'dark brown' of the father was associated with his serious demeanour, gloom and maturity, while the black of the daughter was associated with her rebellious side, her fascination for 'Goth' culture and heavy metal rock music.

Repeatedly and vehemently, the father had objected to his daughter's penchant for black clothing and room decorations. However, when both of them saw the likeness between their selected colours and some of the clothing and shoe images they had associated with that colour, they were able to begin a dialogue and even joke about their similar personalities. Being more relaxed, they could also dialogue more calmly than ever before about ways to honour their differences.

My reason for bringing this colour exercise into the family therapy setting was to relax the participants by helping them experience their playful, creative side, but also to provide a metaphorical vehicle for family members to recognise and accept the ways they resemble and differ from one another. This 'colourful' opening provided the context for just such a therapeutic discussion.

Contours of the Self: Dialogues with the Multifaceted 'I' Voices   *Monica Suswin*

toolek 2

300 4 3

I am not able to impart the meaning of this message to you

I am here to pass on that which has been assigned to me.

I am (Geraldine)

This curious message is the vital information, imprinted on the surface of a red post, written down by Geraldine on a walk across the Ashdown Forest. She had taken on its voice as first person – the 'I' voice – as part of an afternoon workshop:

> Instead of being a bright red painted post of wood as my appearance first suggests, I am actually a shallow slice of metal, so if you look at me from different points of view I change shape. (Geraldine)

Through this voice Geraldine captures something of the nature of being human – this *wooden* post as seen from a distance is in fact something quite different. Later, at home, she developed her voices: 'The following day I felt peaceful and euphoric. I felt a heightened awareness of much more space in which to be oneself.'

The exercise explores and unfolds our inner lives through finding the 'I' voice of things or natural elements in the outer world – the metaphorical outer reflecting aspects of the inner experience.

I start and end the workshops from a studio at the top of our garden; space is limited – five or six people is a comfortable number. People are surprised at the timeless quality of the four-hour session and the quickly formed intimacy of a small group. The aim is to run a monthly workshop with new and old faces but to keep each workshop as an experience in itself. Participants tend to be new to the concept of using writing as a self-reflective tool; writing experience varies as does involvement in personal development. My own background is in both writing and psychotherapy. I try to have a reasonably thorough telephone conversation at the initial contact to explain the point of the work and get a little background on those wishing to attend. This is important so that expectations are defined from the beginning – here will not be the place to write a sonnet! But the real excitement of the group experience is always an unknown quantity – that's what makes it vibrant and enticing.

The exercise
A walk with our notebooks, stopping several times – at each stop, I ask everyone to focus on an aspect of the natural surroundings, or anything at all within view, and to describe this thing with close observation. We do

this three or four times. After the final observation, people choose one, and write from the 'I' perspective.

The fictional 'I am' voice is often explored playfully but held on 'the level of art rather than psychology', as Paul Matthews advocates in *Sing Me the Creation* (1994).

The dialogues

The exercise now goes one step further. It has to be said that it may not suit everyone's imaginative process but, if it works, we create a psychodrama. From the newly discovered 'I' voices, we talk to each other and continue our walk. This needs to be explained clearly or confusion sets in. People need to try and stay in character; this is not necessarily easy. Fritz Perls, who evolved Gestalt therapy (a complex sytem that promotes personal growth through greater awareness of the whole person), speaks of creativity and fantasy 'working when something comes out of the being in touch with what is here and now' (Perls 1971, p.54).

As we walk people come together and part at will, or join in other conversations. However, there is no pressure to join in the dialogues; people can walk in silence if they choose. Amber wrote: 'I did try to avoid getting into conversation yet got into the familiar trap of being polite and joining in.' And Sarah made the point: 'There is vulnerability in the exercise – in trying to communicate with someone who doesn't want to talk to me, I might feel rejected or that I've got it wrong. Here is an exercise which you can enter into or not. This makes for an uneven experience. Can it work?'

This is exactly where the line between therapeutic input and the writing as process treads a delicate path into feelings and how one handles them in this kind of workshop. There is time for reflective writing after the walk and sharing. It does require each individual to take responsibility for their feelings and to feel comfortable and safe with their sharing. My responsibility as leader is to create the boundaries and safety margins in the space and to work within the limits of my own expertise.

Dr Jim Gomersall, who was a senior lecturer at Sheffield University's Department of Psychiatry, believed most practitioners in psychotherapy were lifelong students – the same could be said of this newly developing profession:

> The student needs personal life experience; they should have not
> suffered too much but not suffered too little and healed through
> some form of therapeutic relationship in the broadest definition

of the word. They need professional training in meeting people off the street who are coming for help and to do their best for them with the resources they have. (personal communication)

Example of dialogue: An Oak Sapling and a Slow-Down Sign
Dawn and I entered into conversation with unexpected fun. She was an oak sapling. I was a Slow-Down sign. 20 mph.

Oak sapling:	My branches stretch upwards. My roots grow deep into the earth. I grow slowly.
Slow-Down sign:	Twenty miles an hour is a slow speed. That's the speed I tell people to slow down to.
Oak:	That's too fast for me.
Sign:	Is it? What's slow for you?
Oak:	Ooh – a millimetre or two a day.
Sign:	That's slow.

'I was surprised by the inner strength and calm I felt,' Dawn said. 'I felt free and light and serene. I stepped out of my unquiet mind.'

Example of leaving mid-way through workshop
Amber took on the role of 'garden bench' and wondered: 'Who will sit with [*sic*] me?' However, after the walk, she decided to leave: 'The dialogues tapped straight into where I am at in my life and touched some tender vulnerable spots. I did not want to expose my stuff but that evening I did share my writing with a friend who I felt totally safe with.' Three days later Amber had an individual session. It is true to say that without having come to the workshop Amber would not have been able to leave, and by asserting this need to go she made sure she wasn't sat upon – if we are to understand the true 'I' role of a bench. Despite leaving, Amber made connections both with her friend *and* me and also explored another side of herself later wishing to be 'a leaf happy to be blowing in the wind'.

It was Sarah who had chosen to be 'that yellow leaf – perfectly formed. I left the branch – I drifted – now I am perfectly balanced on the grass. I am an independent leaf – solitary but not alone. I am just as I am.'

Separately both Geraldine and Sarah have come to an acceptance of the Gestalt, the wholeness of themselves in the moment, through identifying with and giving voice to the object in the outer world they have chosen. For them this reflection from outer to inner expression touched a deep acceptance of the self – the underpinning of all the contours of ourselves.

Meet Your Writer Exercise   *Claire Williamson*

Pablo Neruda, in his poem 'We are Many' (1972, p.3), describes the difficulty of deciding on which aspect of the self to 'settle' when each part of us is demanding to be heard. The idea of this exercise is to stop and think and meet the writer part of ourselves. This exercise can be approached internally, externally or both.

External method

Think about the idea of putting on your writer's mask. You might like to draw your mask first. Try describing what the mask looks like and what its colours and patterns represent. Here are some questions you can ask yourself: Do I need my ears, eyes, mouth, nose when I write? What happens behind the mask? Where do I go? What does the mask say to other people?

Internal method

Sit down and write spontaneously. Imagine you are peeling away the layers of your skin and flesh to reveal your writer. Where in the body does your writer live? Start to describe how your writer looks and feels. What does its voice sound like? Is it solid or ghostly? Is it childlike, adult or both? Try and have a dialogue with your writer. Ask it what it needs and how it feels.

The idea behind this exercise is to acquaint yourself with your writer. Think about its needs and whether they are being met. Are their needs unreasonable? Are you being unreasonable with your writer? Be a friend to your writer, so that you can compromise and work together and allow yourself time to be creative and part of the world.

Critic Tango: A Workshop on the Inner Critic
River Wolton

If you seek to tango or tangle with the Inner Critic, beware! Your own Inner Critic will leap into the fray: 'Can you really do this? Who do you think you are? Call yourself a writer...a workshop leader...a valid human being?' Such questions assailed me when I ran a workshop on the Inner Critic (hereafter referred to as the 'Critic') in April 2003, for members of Lapidus. Perhaps my inner critical voices were heightened by the pressure of working with a peer group of experienced writers, many of whom teach writing for a living. By the time the workshop arrived I was in the full swing of a Critic Attack, coupled with rage and despair at the US/UK invasion of Iraq. The Critic that emerged in this atmosphere was merciless. The workshop began with a warm-up using Natalie Goldberg's 'writing practice' technique. In response to the question 'How is the Critic operating in your life right now?' I wrote:

> I am an amalgam of genders, battleships and chessboard squares. I know my precise areas of operation, I creep in and savage my way out. I'm frightened you want to do away with me, that's why I have this big gun between my legs. And I have to keep blasting away in case you see me and my thin skin, my soft underbelly. I am so soft really, that's the secret, I'm really rather easy to blow away. (River Wolton)

Since addressing the Critic can heighten its powers and may lead directly into traumatic memories, I suggested to participants that they bring a gentle curiosity to the writing and approach the subject with as much lightness as possible. Several of the exercises involved stepping into the Critic's shoes and writing in its voice, in order to uncover its origins, as in this piece by Miriam Halahmy.

> *Critic:* Her mother laughed when she was ten, 'Ha! We all wrote poetry!' Approval of her writing from her mother was essential. She never got it and so the door was left open for me. I padded in stinking from the jungle and have stayed here ever since.

What emerged was a strong connection between the personal and the political. Participants wrote about childhood messages that originated in racism, anti-Semitism or bullying. Writers from black, Jewish and working-class backgrounds wrote about being told, directly and indirectly, 'Keep your head down', 'Don't draw attention to yourself', 'Don't get too big for your boots'. For many of us the Critic evolved out of protective intentions (such as parents' warnings to children vulnerable to prejudice, bullying and disappointment) but had become an immense block to creative development, self-perception and confidence. I was struck by the resonances with education and religion; at times our Critics epitomised a version of patriarchal fundamentalism. Anne Maney's poem begins:

A Tall Black Hat by Anne Maney

Bells, high metallic chimes outside the heavy door.
His voice, low and resonant, from up there down to my level.
like a deep-toned bell from a tower.
No smile, exactly. A folding of the skin around grey eyes –
the colour of the sea he dreams of.
The hands have not done manual work,
they are long-fingered and the skin fits firmly and smoothly.
He does not touch me…

It is particularly tricky for writers to use writing as a means for uncovering the Critic. The Critic thrives in educational and literary settings. 'Writer's block' is the Critic in action. Some writers may believe they don't have a Critic but they would certainly recognise the repetitive thought loops that were common for the workshop participants: 'Not good/clever/prolific/original/funny/serious/worthwhile/daring …enough (or at all).' With some adjustments these internal messages can be applied to anything we attempt as human beings. Coming up against them can be overwhelming. In the workshop we focused on the five senses, and homed in on precise details, to bear witness to the Critic's character, actions and motivations.

Inner Critic by Joanna Ezekiel

I am a locked gate
in front of that detached house
in Chigwell. The jeep in the drive.
Ring on the harsh bell.
Pass my pillars of stone.
The smell of gin. Piranhas
in the swimming pool.
My PhD from Cambridge, framed.
The wallpaper the colour
of the cool cream of reason.
Breathe it all in.
Then try to exhale.

In *The Shaman's Body* (1993) Arny Mindell describes how the blocking nature of symptoms or inner voices can be counteracted by amplifying the 'Ally' or potentially helpful aspect of a difficulty. We began to explore this idea, by writing a conversation between the Critic and a Mediator who wants to find out how the Critic can be helpful. At this point we were pushed for time, and the interesting dialogues that emerged merited more space for development.

Mediator:	What do you want from [Miriam]?
Critic:	To stop her as soon as she starts to raise that pen from the page.
Mediator:	Is that all?
Critic:	Yes.
Mediator:	Really, isn't there something more?
Critic:	I want standards. Not the impossible benchmark of her family. But the standards by which we measure quality. Does the writing work? Have you tried your best? Could you rephrase, reflect more deeply, widen research? Standards for God's sake!
Mediator:	So why do you try so hard to stop her?
Critic:	That's my job.
Mediator:	How could you be more useful?
Critic:	Can't.
Mediator:	Oh come on. Course you can.
Critic:	Let her win sometimes. Become an ally. Let her see that I have a role to play in her work, but of course, she must stay in control.

(Miriam Halahmy)

The workshop participants devised questions for their Critics: 'What do you want? How could you be useful to me? How could we work together? What is your wisdom? What is your secret?' By this point we were developing a sense of enquiry, able to stand back from the battle and observe exactly how it was being fought. Many of us were surprised to discover that there were alternatives other than destroying the Critic or being destroyed by it.

After the workshop a sense of achievement mingled with the familiar nagging of internal criticism, but participants' comments indicated that we had broken new ground. With the hindsight of 18 months, the menace running through the writing seems stark, and the connection between inner and outer violence even sharper. The quality of the writing that emerged reflects the vitality that can be present when we tackle the Critic head-on, affirming my belief that the Critic's energy can be recycled to hone and sharpen. The tango is a dance of passion and intensity performed with a thorny rose between the teeth, but we do not always have to let the Critic take the lead.

CHAPTER 8

Who am I?

Edited by Gillie Bolton

This one brief question is central to our work. All the chapters of *Writing Works*, in a way, explore the vital question 'Who am I?' Curiosity about this question is not restricted to those in need of therapy, counselling or self-help. Its self-illuminating genuine examination, however, is restricted to brave explorers willing to pass beyond the safe frontiers of their own well-known personal world. Helping people to question themselves, come face to face with themselves, has to be undertaken cautiously. This chapter's writers are trustworthy guides. Their exercises and workshops are carefully designed as guiding maps for adventurers, and to offer support and succour on the way.

It's not so much *what* you do but *how* you do it that can give writers the confidence to explore themselves. The exercises River Wolton gave an ME (myalgic encephalomyelitis) support group were very simple, yet enabled them to trust the process and themselves. They felt in control of the writing process, and that their writing was their own to do with whatever they wanted.

The other chapter authors used specific, very carefully worded exercises to help people towards this sense of enquiry and confident ownership. Irmeli Laitinen helped her mental health clients gain more agency over their own treatment with carefully supported structured diary work. Geri Giebel Chavis enabled her psychotherapeutic clients to find out what it was they felt, why and how, through creating simple short pieces. Relating to writing which they came to see as poems helped them to perceive who they were and who they wanted to be. Steven Weir, Debbie McCulliss and Annette Ecuyeré Lee's client groups were all students or peers. They indicate, however, how the work they describe can be adapted for clients or patients. They use careful pacing so that participants are not faced with too much too soon, and judicious timing of the sharing of writing to help bring material out gradually into the relatively safe environment of the group.

Structured Diaries for Depressed Women's Self-Help Groups   *Irmeli Laitinen*

One day in January 1995 my workmate, Tanja, and I were having a team meeting, discussing our clients in the adult mental health office in Helsinki. I still remember that afternoon even though it was over ten years ago. The Finnish landscape was covered with white snow. It looked romantic outside; inside me I felt the heaviness of my workload. Tanja and I were sharing our feelings, thoughts and concerns: it did not take us long to realise that we had so many women who were depressed and who had been visiting our office for many, many years. I was feeling kind of desperate and asked, 'Do you think we are doing something wrong here? It doesn't seem like we are helping these women so much.'

These women had been coming to us for many years; their treatment was called a 'contact hour' in which there was no therapeutic intervention. In my mind, these contact hours were going nowhere. It was frustrating for us and especially for them. Knowing that we had a long waiting list made the situation difficult for us. How could we respond to their needs effectively?

Tanja and I discussed what we would like to happen if we were in their shoes, so to speak. Immediately, I said that I would like to have a women's group where I could share my feelings and problems with other women. And there the Women and Depression Project (WDP) started. It involved a short-term, therapeutic intervention to help depressed women. Through this work, I created a guided self-help programme and published a handbook.

Our first group began in March with 12 women. While the group included self-help strategies, the whole process encouraged women to learn how to help themselves out of the depression or at least to become skilled in accepting or managing it. We understood self-help as individual self-care, based on individuals' own knowledge and experience. In the WDP groups, this knowledge was gathered by diaries. The first self-help step was for members to be knowledgeable about and name their problems in their diaries. Naming and making their problems part of their consciousness meant they internalised them and had a 'psychological relationship' with them. They started to own their own problems. The next step was for them to engage with interventions for change.

Topic-focused group sessions were held once a week for ten weeks. During the first group session, each member received her own diary, a list of group topics and dates for the group sessions. Each session began and ended with 'a feeling circle' when each member in turn shared her feelings, to help group members unite and participate better in the group process, and to make the group a safe place for expression of feeling. As the group leader, I began to see changes in these women's lives. They were not so depressed.

We always looked at the women's diaries in the groups. Every week there was a written diary task. The first week's, for example, was to write down a list of problems, pains and unpleasant feelings as well as positive events and successes. Diaries helped their writers become more conscious of what was happening in their everyday lives whether it was perceived as being good or bad. The diary was also a therapeutic and healing tool. I noticed the diaries helped generate a connection in the women to what was unknown in themselves and was becoming conscious (i.e. their unconscious or dreams). I suspected this would happen because I was an advocate of diaries for myself and my friends.

Group members discussed how easy or difficult the tasks were to write down. If a member forgot her diary task, all of us in the group tried to help her. With her, we looked at her forgetfulness from a psychodynamic point of view. We asked if this was how she treated herself. Did she tend to forget herself and her needs? Besides the diary centrepiece there were short papers presented by group facilitators, art work, open discussions on the week's topic either in a big or small group, video presentations and relaxation exercises.

Given the many different ways to work on one's problems, these women began to accept that they were different from one another. The group strategies helped them to respect themselves and the way they worked on their problems. There were some women who mainly wrote in their diaries and/or did art work: they did not participate very much in group discussions. There were other women who could hardly write anything in their diaries but were very active in group discussions. To look at how differently women used their diaries as a therapeutic tool, I counted the pages: the longest was 395 and the shortest, five. I always felt the diary was a mirroring tool for these women's inner lives. It enabled them to understand better their depression and to recognise how they reacted to it in their everyday lives.

From my memorable winter afternoon with Tanja, the WDP with a diary group centrepiece began. Since then, there have been many groups based on the WDP group method. Before I moved to England, I facilitated 14 groups for 140 women in Finland in places such as family therapy centres, alcohol treatment centres, women's therapy centres and university counselling services. For me, it has included some of the most important therapeutic work in my life. Long live diaries!

Bursting Free: Writing and ME   *River Wolton*

In 2002 I was invited to work with an ME (myalgic encephalomyelitis) self-help group that uses creativity and art to help recovery and healing from the extreme fatigue that characterises the disease. Over the year I ran four writing sessions, the first two focusing on the experience of having ME, and the last two using real and remembered family photographs.

In the introductions to the sessions, my emphasis on 'Whatever you write is right. You can't write the wrong thing!' (borrowed from Gillie Bolton) seemed particularly helpful. Other tips included:

> This writing is for you, you don't have to share it if you don't want to. Once you start writing keep the pen moving, even if you write lists or repeat yourself. Don't plan, just write down whatever comes into your head. Keep breathing!

Each session started with a warm-up – for example, 'Being here today I feel...' or 'Writing here today reminds me of...' or 'I want my words to...'. These starting points were drawn from the writing practice method of Natalie Goldberg (1986, 1991).

> I want my words to express what I feel beautifully, succinctly, elegantly, movingly, inspiringly. I want them to move people so much that people with ME, and all people with disabilities, get treated write [*sic*]. I want my words to educate people, including me. I want my words to forge connections between us isolated in our little foetal sacs. I want my words to burst the sacs, the liquid to run out into the sea, us to step out alive and free to embrace each other. The Great Gig in the sky – Passion. All the passion I ever felt expressed in one screaming song, rising and dying and falling and rising again. (Marie King)

Much of the writing expressed the disconnection and isolation caused by ME. There was also great sadness at the losses brought by chronic illness and the ways it had been misunderstood by family, friends and doctors.

> It's easier to pass for well. Some people who know something about ME are sympathetic. Eyebrows go up in 'Ahhh, what a shame.' Faces may be blank because they don't know what it is, what it means to my life, even if they've heard the name. My body is not separate from the environment, and it has been polluted – food, air, water, capitalism. I think this, I don't say it very often. It helps to feel that my body, my disease is not isolated, just me, but I am part of the living environment, many people and plants and animals are affected by disease, the degraded environment. I want to take the mystery out of ME. Sometimes I am in denial, just to get by and to focus on other things in my life. (Gill Owens)

In writing and discussion, the group explored the tension between wanting the illness to be taken seriously and wanting to be validated as a complex person, not just 'someone with ME'. We used an exercise on identity from Schneider and Killick (1998), making lists under the headings 'I am…' and 'I am not…', and then choosing one from each list for the start of a longer piece.

Football Fan by *Liz*

I am a Football Fan,
a Wigan Latic fanatic
four forty-five Saturday,
the footie scores come in,
listen on your 'tranny' while you leave the ground.
I've bought the shirt
and a bobble hat too,
it's great being part of a crowd
when illness sets you apart.
Have a good moan
a cup of coffee from your flask at half time,
remember to wear your thickest socks
and two pair.
Sing up for Wigan

Ooh Ahh
Ooooh Ahh
Oooh to be a Wig – on – ar
I wish I could go every week,
the ups and downs
my Soap not on TV.

The theme of death and dying emerged strongly, and I began to see how the prejudice and misunderstandings that surround people with chronic illness might arise from their involuntary role in confronting the rest of us with our mortality and transitory able-bodiedness. One participant quoted a friend who had survived ME and cancer and had said that the cancer was easier to deal with, partly because other people were more sympathetic and knew how to react. We wrote and talked about the gains and losses brought by illness, and the 'wisdom' learned through having ME. Several participants felt that these discussions were as important as the writing itself. I often left more leeway for talking than I usually would, because the group functioned as a vital point of social contact, especially when participants were spending much of their time at home or in bed.

> My ME is a very wise, old person, about 90, a sage with infinite knowledge and wisdom, Merlin. Long white hair, long earth-coloured robes. Merlin says, 'Listen to me. Do it slowly. Stop. Don't do that. Do this. Do it now. Do it in one month. See – now you know. You did it wrong then – you have to pay. It's only right. You'll find out.' Most of the time I don't see Merlin but sometimes he appears like a thought, here and gone in a trice. He's beckoning me down a lane. This is my path and I have to follow it. (Marie King)

I wanted to offer the group a taste of reflective writing and the resources it might bring for well-being, and to provide some perspectives on the 'demon' of illness, using ideas from Gestalt, from Mindell's *The Shaman's Body* (1993) and from *The Alchemy of Illness* by Kat Duff (1993), a writer and counsellor who has lived with chronic illness. As the workshops progressed, my own 'blind spots' about ME surfaced; for example, I thought that photographs might provide a gentle way into exploring the experience of being ill. In fact, the process of looking through and choosing old photos was intensely painful for some group members, because it was a concrete reminder of what had been lost. I sometimes over-estimated energy levels or mistimed pacing, and it was important to remind the group not to try too hard and to stay relaxed. The group was all-female, by accident rather than design, and in writing about photographs one question that emerged was this: who are we as women if we are not well enough to nurture, take care of others and be constantly on the go?

> Look at how I am in the picture. Cuddled up to Grandma. And for extra security I'm hanging on to my 'Lee', my blanket which smells sweet, like a faraway biscuit.

> Because I am a little girl no one will say this is strange, instead it will be seen as me doing what girls/women do – engaging in the pattern of nurturing/being nurtured. No one is going to help me become independent. In fact, they will subtly and not so subtly discourage it. Instead they will encourage me to be soft and dependent, because in some complicated way that takes care of them; and very quickly I will start directly taking care of them too. I'm going to enjoy this and yet I'll also be building myself a trap. Making myself feel important and worth something, yes, but their dependence will be such it will be terribly hard to leave, to move on, to grow, to be a separate person, feeling separate, being perceived as separate.

> And I'll spend many years finding it terribly hard to believe I'm worth something even when I'm *not* nurturing or being nurtured. I get little early practice. I start late. I'm too dependent on relationships. This saps my strength. (Anna Ravetz)

We explored real and imaginary photos and wrote about the strengths and unique qualities that we could see in them. In particular whether our past 'selves' had any message for our present 'selves':

> The woman in the photo says: be happy, have fun, take happiness wherever you can find it, look for it, go after it, grab it by the scruff of the neck – it's yours. Happiness is there somewhere. Don't shy away from it. Even in the most unpromising circumstances you can find something to make you happy. And when you've found it, experience it fully. Let it fill your being while it lasts. (Marie King)

After the writing sessions, the group worked with a graphic designer to bring the words and photographs to life through digital imaging. Although many participants had no previous experience of creative writing or graphic design they described the work as 'very rewarding and inspiring'. The project culminated in an exhibition of text and images that toured in community centres and local libraries. It was a powerful evocation of the experience of ME and a testimony to the ability of creative expression to inform and change perception. In a real sense it forged connections and broke open the 'foetal sacs' of isolation. Working with the group altered my own perspective on illness and was an enriching opportunity. We continue to work together on other writing projects.

With many thanks to the group and the participants whose work is quoted. Some names have been changed by request. The project was funded by National Lottery 'Awards for All' and the Abbey National Community Partnership. There are over 240,000 sufferers of ME (myalgic encephalo-myelitis), also known as CFS (chronic fatigue syndrome), and diagnosed as PVFS (post viral fatigue syndrome) in the UK. Debilitating fatigue is a common symptom, but is also an inadequate description of the illness and its effects. See March (1998) and the Action for ME website (www.afme.org.uk).

Motivating for Success   *Steven Weir*

My turn had come around to run a workshop for a local group of writers interested in writing for personal development. The workshop was to be held mid-January, so I began to think about the sort of issues that we tend to face at that time of year. The recurring theme, common to us all, I decided, related to motivation. After the promises of brighter days we make to ourselves in January, we tend to slip away from our best intentions by the middle of the month.

The workshop allowed an hour and a half of writing time and was attended by about six people. As I would be inviting participants to explore not only a goal that was important to them, but also the often intensely personal motivations for wanting to achieve it, I made it clear at the beginning that there would be no expectation for anyone to read their work.

I began the workshop with a 'free-flow' warm-up exercise. This was to ensure that the group left the cold night outside and were able to focus on the inner world of their aspirations.

I asked the group to define a goal that was important to them. This could be in the form of a New Year's resolution or a longer-standing goal. The goal was to be contained within one sentence and be in wholly positive form. The reason for this is that a goal of, for example, 'not failing' can only be achieved after understanding what failure would mean and then moving away from it. This sets up an inner conflict and wastes energy getting clear about what we don't want.

Having established a goal, we attached a time frame for achieving it. I asked the group, if necessary, to break it down into something they could envisage happening within about six months. We then imagined that the goal had already been realised, writing about how our 'future selves' felt about themselves and the world around them. I asked the participants to write about whether we looked different in any way, sounded different or carried ourselves more confidently. How did it feel to have achieved this goal? How did other people respond to us? What was our day like? Our environment?

Exploring all the ways in which the dream makes a difference does two things. First, it clarifies whether we really want to reach that target, or whether we need to redefine it in some way. Second, it helps the dream to take on more substance as we explore all of the ripple effect.

Having got really clear about the goal and the difference that achieving it would make, we explored, through our writing, our reasons for wanting this goal and the things that might get in our way.

For the second part of the evening, I wanted to draw out an experience of success that each member of the group had previously achieved. To encourage the members to become fully associated with their own achievement, I asked them to write about a goal they'd accomplished or a success they'd had, however small it might have been. What had motivated them to act when they first began – were they trying to decrease their pain or increase their pleasure in some way? What kept them going when it became an uphill struggle? What kinds of things were they saying to themselves to keep motivated?

To bring the first two parts of the workshop together, the group applied what they had learnt about their own motivation during the second part to the goal they identified at the beginning. Participants wrote about how the strength of their motivation would help them to overcome the barriers that might get in their way, getting as clear as possible about what they would say, do or be which would keep them on track. Last, everyone identified one action they needed to take and made an agreement with themselves about when and where they would do it.

At the end of the writing time, the energy in the room had shifted. Everyone was contemplative yet buzzing. We all had a plan in place to begin to move more confidently towards our goal.

One or two people shared their experience of the workshop process, without going into details about their own work. Most had come away with a clearer and deeper understanding of their dream and what it meant to them as well as an agreement (with themselves) about the next steps to take. Several months later one participant commented about a chain of events set in motion by the exercise, which had refocused her energy on completing her book.

The steps involved in this workshop are quite similar to creative visualisation, which is a technique I have used for many years. I've always found it an invaluable way of accessing the power of my imagination. However, breaking the process down in written form has the advantage of giving us the space to really explore our ideas. By giving ourselves permission to write whatever comes into our minds, we often uncover new and exciting aspects of ourselves, and can see them more clearly as they stare back at us from the page.

Systems like neurolinguistic programming (Robbins 2001) and Kahuna, the Hawaiian shamanic tradition (King 1990), have influenced my work, giving me the tools to explore the inner landscapes more confidently.

Two Vignettes   *Geri Giebel Chavis*

Body wisdom and voice

A single 30-year-old woman gymnast and dancer studying to be a massage therapist had been seeing me in 50-minute psychotherapeutic sessions every two weeks for approximately six months at a large psychiatric clinic. Having been focusing on her strained relationship with her mother and with identity, self-esteem and relationship issues, she trusted her body but was struggling to find her 'voice' as a speaker and writer. She was very anxious about being what she called 'inarticulate' and 'unorganised' in speaking both within and outside our sessions. She recalled her exasperation and guilt over her mother's lack of 'voice', a limitation she associated with her mother's sadness and helplessness as a single parent. Very aware of an inner 'gap' or empty space, she believed this resulted from never being asked by her mother how she felt or what she thought.

During our work together, she was attempting to fill that void through discovering her own 'woman wisdom'. By the fourteenth session, she expressed, with trepidation, her desire to capture in writing some of the discoveries made during therapy. As a preliminary to the writing activity, I invited her to use body language to depict her feelings and thoughts, and then I suggested she use a large sheet of paper at home with room for the 'silences' as well as the words. She indicated at the following session that her fears had prevented her from writing; we addressed her assumptions about my expectations, and I suggested she either write or choose not to write and not tell me either way.

This seemed to free her of a burden, and she proceeded to articulate aloud important aspects of her truth. Without her realising, I took on the role of scribe as I listened to her detail the link between her present-day anxiety within her apartment and her past experience of moving:

> silently like a cat on soundless feet
> who saw lots and had wisdom.

Her flow of words also included the desire to be 'a lioness with a roar'.

When I read aloud the words she had instinctively voiced in the form of a poem and presented this writing to her, she was amazed, exhilarated and embarrassed. Although she feared she would later judge her work, she did take it home and even elaborated on it. She described herself as 'moving stealthily, like a cat, around a deep, large core of her mother's grief' and noted how her present day 'tiptoeing' to avoid disturbing downstairs neighbours evoked memories of her mother's 'reservoir of sadness'. She continued to describe, in writing, how her present-day dancing and gymnastic skill enabled her to 'walk flat on the ground' instead of 'tiptoeing' as a gymnast and how she was even getting used to the 'stamping' and 'roaring' she was expected to do in her dance routine.

Through her short writing, this young woman not only began to trust her capacity to be articulate in a variety of school and social settings, but also affirmed her recent attempts to free her body from the long-held visceral reactions to her mother's burdens.

Imaging the self in and out of role

A 32-year-old man came to my private practice to discuss his anxiety, frustration and lack of assertiveness in his four-year marriage. He was exploring his identity as a husband and whether or not he wanted to stay married. During our fourth session together, I invited him to write his definition of self as a husband and then to imagine himself as not a husband by using the following two sentence stems:

'When I am a husband...' and 'If I were not a husband...'

Here is what he wrote:

When I am a husband,
I am a wife-supplicant,
A downtrodden, hunched-over man
Suffocating.

If I were not a husband,
I would have solitude,
The absence of guilt,
Freedom to do what I want
Without consequence,
Freedom to explore who I am.

This poem functioned as a catalyst for a fruitful discussion of major feelings, self-defeating behaviour patterns and previously unrecognised options for expressing the self.

Creating Your Mission Statement for Life and Work
Debbie McCulliss

Have you ever been drawn to pick a book up after seeing it a number of times on the bookshelf? For months each time I walked out of my home office, my eyes were drawn to *The Path: Creating Your Mission Statement for Work and for Life* by Laurie Beth Jones (1996), a gift from a work colleague. After repeated episodes of shaking my head, I finally picked it up and looked through it in June 2002.

That summer I decided to recruit a group of four other women by word of mouth. We were all in our forties and early fifties, two worked full-time, one worked part-time and two were students. Each had two or three children, the youngest being 12 years old and the oldest being 24 years old at the time. Before the class started three of us felt we were on the right path and the other two felt they were having a crisis of purpose.

We met for two and a half to three hours five times over the course of a month and a half in my home. The goal was to develop a brief, succinct and focused statement of purpose that can be used to initiate, evaluate and refine all life's activities based on the reading and exercises in the book. Other objectives included:

- to facilitate others to develop their own mission statement
- to identify 11 false assumptions about mission statements
- to discuss three qualities of a good mission statement
- to practise exercises that help one discover what is truly important to oneself.

Other plans for the class included:

- to provide thought-provoking questions
- to facilitate group dynamics
- to encourage sharing of answers during class
- to encourage feedback from others.

To begin exploring our personal mission we reflected on the following questions:

1. What is your reason for getting up and going to work in the morning? Do you have a clear sense of purpose?

2. Do you love what you are doing so much that time flies and you feel extraordinarily alive?

3. Are you working hard but not finding meaning and fulfilment?

4. Are you unclear about what is important or what to do next?

5. Are your natural strengths not being used effectively?

6. Are you serving humankind, somehow making the world a better place? (Questions from Higher Awareness 2001)

Ralph Waldo Emerson says:

> The purpose of life is not to be happy. It is to be useful, to be honourable, to be compassionate, and to have it make some difference that you have lived and lived well. (Quoted in Leider 1994, p.40)

Laurie Beth Jones says:

> A mission statement acts as both a harness and a sword –
> harnessing you to what is true about one's life, and cutting
> away all that is false… A good mission statement will be
> inspiring, exciting, clear, and engaging. It will be specific to you
> and your particular enthusiasms, gifts and talents. (Jones 1996,
> pp.xvii, 65)

It will benefit others. All of your activities should flow from and relate back
to your mission. Mission statements can change.

> Sustaining your personal mission means staying on the path that
> belongs to you, and this requires continuous evaluation and
> renewal of the journey. The ability to evaluate your journey is
> critical to staying on course. (Hudson 1999, p.85)

Evaluation of the class included:

- attendance
- participant participation in each class
- participant evaluation
- self-evaluation.

In guiding others I found the process insightful, meaningful and worthwhile. Some shed tears while others said, 'Oh yeah.' Lessons that I was
reminded of throughout the classes included: it is always about the process
not the destination; a knowing of what we teach is what we need to learn
ourselves and to dare to go deeper each time.

> Once we know and align with our uniqueness and know what
> gives us meaning, we are creating a soul connection. This
> enables us to experience more love, peace, joy, freedom, service,
> understanding and fulfilment. (Higher Awareness 2001)

The experience was positive for all in the class!

Personal Heraldic Coat of Arms   *Annette Ecuyeré Lee*

I used this exercise with a ten-credit, lifelong learning course run by
the University of Wales Aberystwyth, on creative writing for personal
development. The group met fortnightly for four hours with time split
between guided exercises, discussion, group work and tutorials. Half the
participants had been on courses with me before and there was a mix of
writing abilities. I facilitate writing groups in many different situations and

use this exercise in most of them; from induction day exercises with new students in university to personal development sessions with business people and creative writers.

I developed it from an opening exercise at a PGCE (Post Graduate Certificate of Education) course I attended. The lecturer, Simon Evans, used the shield with the drawing and show and tell parts as a 'getting to know you' exercise and I have added the writing section as a way to encourage openings for personal development.

The exercise revolved around participants producing a coat of arms and a personal motto to go with it. I gave them all a sheet of paper – at least A3 in size. I also only provided coloured pencils, wax crayons and large marker pens to encourage boldness and to prevent them becoming worried or precious about their drawings.

I drew a large template of an heraldic shield/coat of arms for them to copy which I then divided into four sections labelled Hobbies/Interests; Family/Social; Education; Occupation/Career.

In each section I asked them to put in images or symbols to represent whatever is relevant to their lives. No words are allowed in the shield – only images – and although this can cause some initial resistance from those who feel they cannot draw, I have never had anyone who did not have a go and actually enjoy the process.

A banner at the bottom of the shield was for them to produce a motto or their philosophy in life for themselves. This produced a range from 'be happy' to 'if nothing else it's not boring'.

After approximately 20 minutes they were all encouraged to go through their drawings and mottos. This really lightened the group as well as bringing them together as they found out bits about each other.

I asked them to choose one image from any area of the shield they wanted to develop, and asked them to draw up a plan, or a mind map, exploring their chosen piece and then to write this up as a fictional character – not as themselves.

Some group members were sceptical about writing the piece from another person's viewpoint and were genuinely surprised at the outcome. They gained insights about themselves and enjoyed the freedom that using a character allowed them in developing their chosen topic.

Edith Thomas was particularly delighted with her response, although it was the group and tutorial discussions that helped her find the greatest insights. When I first taught Edith she was very new to the art of writing and every attempt was followed by apologies for her lack of ability. Since then she has continued, quite fruitfully, and has stopped apologising for herself and her work. Attempts at other creative activities have also met with success; she has found a new self-respect and is now confident enough to not only encourage others around her, but has also led a group of her own within her church.

Edith's story

'Audrey you have made a complete recovery. You're better. I know it has been a long illness and for that reason it will be a while before you feel 100 per cent fit. My advice is to go out and meet new people, learn a new skill, find a new hobby.'

'Thank you Doctor for all your care over these last months. But don't you think I need a tonic or pain killers?'

Doctor Jones shook his head and smiled his goodbye smile. Audrey left the surgery slowly. She felt so tired and depressed. She didn't want to do anything but perhaps the doctor's advice would help her…

The next Monday evening found Audrey outside the village hall shivering with fright. Doctor's orders alone had brought her there. She was about to run away when three young people piled out of a car just by her and swept her into the hall. They were laughing and talking in such a friendly way that she stopped shivering and looked about her with interest.

There was no dreaded audition. They just accepted that she was an alto and that she could read music. It was as well they did not ask her how well she could read music! The first piece they practised was familiar and she was able to let go and sing with delight. What an evening! So many enthusiastic people surging round her and singing beside her, she was uplifted beyond her wildest imaginings. She was so grateful to her doctor for his good advice.

In her reflections on her writing Edith commented:

It seemed odd to me that my subconscious could see my mothering years as a long illness! It is true that my creativity only emerged during those years as the odd knitted garment and dresses for my offspring. Did I really have to wait for 'authority' or the doctor figure to give me permission to do what I wanted to do?

She also commented that she 'was very interested in the different approaches that the other members of the group took – we differed quite startlingly'.

The exercise is non-threatening, can be guided easily by the tutor, and is also great fun. What must be accepted though is that it can bring in some unexpected emotions for the writers, but I tend to find that following the session with a group discussion or an individual tutorial deals with any issues that can arise.

CHAPTER 9

Life's Journey

Edited by Gillie Bolton

Where am I in myself now? Where have I been? And where might I be in the future? These are all questions which obsess most of us. Writing is an appropriate way of trying to overcome some of the blocks in our minds which readily prevent open examination of such vital questions. Like Chapter 8, 'Who am I?', all the chapters in this book could be said to be exploring these issues. But whereas they come at the questions metaphorically or at a slant, these workshops tackle them head on.

Rose Flint's deceptively simple, yet powerfully locating exercise for exploring 'where I am now' would help anyone to gain clarity about their current mood and thinking. Being more observant and aware of surroundings and personal response can help people to be more at ease in and gain more pleasure from their surroundings. I have used an exercise to help professionals gain a clearer picture of themselves in their workplace. I ask them to walk into their work space first thing in the morning, in their minds' eyes. They note down what they see, hear, smell, touch and taste, and then what they think and feel. What they find they've written can be intensely mind-opening. We take so much for granted without thinking: 'Do I like this? Is this what I want?', and, most important, 'What can I change? What do I want to change?' A tiny writing exercise can help people suddenly feel: 'I've never noticed that before and it's wonderful!', or 'I've never before focused on how I hate this every day; now I'm going to change it!'

Locating yourself out of yourself in order to look constructively at your own writing can be illuminating. John Hilsdon very clearly and simply explains how to read a piece of writing as if it was written by someone else. Personal writing involves writers to such an extent that they can become blinkered and not perceive the full effects of their writing, or the impact of images. Writing is always a communication: the first interlocutor is the self.

Personal writers can sometimes be their own sole reader. Rereading one's own explorative expressive writing nearly always has an impact; using a strategy to distance one's reading self from one's writing self can increase this.

Angie Butler describes reminiscence work in a workshop with elderly people writing alongside young children. Reminiscence work, sensitively handled, can offer older people great enjoyment as well as personal benefit. Reminding them of their younger days, it can be a joy to remember loved people who are now deceased, and how things used to be. Reminiscence and life writing can reconnect them positively with themselves in previous times, past events, past ways. Sharing some of these things with younger people can also give them a living view of recent history, and share the wisdom accrued with age and experience.

Jo Monks powerfully uses other arts alongside writing to facilitate a friend's journey. The journey of life is as old a metaphor as storytelling and self-understanding itself. My workshop could be adapted in myriads of ways. One method is to ask people to list (or draw on a long piece of paper) the milestones of their life. Participants can then write more about whichever of these they wish. I often ask people to think of less obvious milestones; these have included 'when I realised I didn't love him any more', rather than 'my divorce', and 'when I went to boarding school'.

First Thing   *Rose Flint*

As poet in residence for the Kingfisher Project, running creative writing workshops in both a city community and hospital, I am constantly meeting new groups of people. Some may be confined to their bed or the ward for a long time; others may live at home and use a variety of community centres; some may be experiencing only a brief hospitalisation. I never really know what to expect from any new group; they are all unique. I always want to base the work I do with them on what they bring to the workshops themselves, rather than what I could impose on them, so beginnings can feel difficult for me. If a group is thoroughly urban they may not appreciate being asked to write about birds, for instance. So over the years I have started to use exercises which are adaptable and relevant at all times.

This exercise is one that will often tell me a great deal about the individual writer. It may tell me about their mood, whether they are depressed or have any capacity for optimism, for instance. It will also give clues to the location they live in. By this I don't mean just the physical environment but how they locate themselves within it, or alongside it. This gives me a sense of their relationship to both their surroundings and to themselves, both mind and body. As a simple list, it is also a very easy piece of writing for anyone to do, and has a good sense of completion. Even group members or the individuals that I work with on a one-to-one basis who say they 'can't write' and are nervous of the idea can do this as well as anyone else. The exercise also signals the start of something for all of us, as I will do it alongside everyone else, which gives them an opportunity to know more about me.

Most exercises provide frameworks for creativity. The idea of framework rather than form is, I think, something of great value to the writer in health care, or indeed the writers who work with any inexperienced groups. Frames do not need to be complex – rather the reverse – and yet they can provide a strong structure for a writer to hold before they are ready to move off into their own spontaneous or responsive writing.

I used this exercise, First Thing This Morning I... in the Spinal Unit, at our very first session. After the usual introductions, I asked them to write – or I scribed – just a simple list:

> First Thing This Morning I saw... I heard... I smelled... I tasted... I touched... I dreamed... (and/or) I thought...

One young man, a tetraplegic with no feeling in his upper body, wrote that he had 'patted a nurse's bum but felt nothing'. A woman who had had a riding accident wrote that she dreamed she 'rode her horse and flew'. The smells and sounds of the early morning ward came very clearly, toast and urine, a kind voice, the clatter of a bin. From this exercise I had gained an immediate and very intimate snapshot of life in the unit, the good and the difficult parts of it, each individual's response to something that was familiar to all.

This 'snapshot' framework can be varied a great deal. Suggesting the same 'senses plus' list in another setting can also provide information of the focused, detailed kind that makes a good poem. Working with mental health service users who were living in their own homes but attending a day/resource centre, another version provided a good take-off point for further poems. This community group was always small, usually three or perhaps five young men. I worked with them over a 12-week period, in an upper room at the day centre. Sometimes we used an hour and a half, sometimes only an hour, depending on their energy. I had asked them to use the same framework of the senses to write about 'the journey from home to here'.

Walking Down the Road

I saw a delighted market researcher
I heard a soft tick direction indicator
I smelled exhausts on the wind
I tasted my blood through my palate
I touched the knurled button
I thought about those times I still can't kill.

This writer found the 'frame' very freeing. He often had confusing and conflicting thoughts, which prevented him from writing. Working with the small detailed canvas of a frame such as this represented a real freedom to explore both feelings and memories.

Who Wrote This?   *John Hilsdon*

Encouraging some of my counselling clients and students to try Peter Elbow's (1998) 'freewriting' technique in recent years (Hilsdon 2004) led me to develop the Who Wrote This? exercise. I first tried it with a group of nursing students who were complaining bitterly that tutors criticised their essay writing but that no one ever taught them how to write. Feeling their frustration, I heard myself saying, 'Well, just for now, forget about how to write. Try seeing what it's like to read instead!' Some eyebrows rose. 'Look – try this,' I said, grabbing a spare chair, the idea still forming in my mind. I had decided to act out a version of a Two Chairs exercise, one commonly used in counselling. Each chair becomes a different aspect of the self, or the self and an imaginary interlocutor.

'First, just be you! Take that essay and give it in.' I reached across and slapped papers down onto the chair next to me. 'And now,' I said, warming to this chance for a bit of comedy, 'sit there yourself.' I moved to the second chair, theatrically grasped the 'essay', peered at it, and then cried imperiously: 'I wonder who wrote this!' There were chuckles in the room. 'And I wonder,' I continued, looking now at the group, 'what it has to say!'

Aside from the cathartic and stress-relieving function of this playful approach, serious creative, therapeutic and/or academic purposes can be addressed in this way. My group of nurses, the ice broken, soon got stuck into the task of reviewing their own writing – playing the parts of writer and reader/tutor, with both hilarious and productive consequences. Reviewing the session, they agreed that being prepared consciously to adopt the role of reader – and moreover, a *critical* reader – when in the 'other' chair was of enormous benefit in helping them to edit and rework their writing. The nurses' main concerns were, first, to ensure they had included what the assignment required and, second, to express themselves clearly and in an appropriate style.

Subsequently I have seen enormous potential for creative and therapeutic work from this exercise. For its full impact, participants need to be willing to question their views of writing and identity – albeit just for the duration of the exercise. Allowing that we cannot really know anything perfectly, there is always more to discover, to understand – there is always a degree of uncertainty about knowledge. If we accept such a view, we open our minds to the possibility of new perceptions, ideas, questions and understandings. From this position, when we engage with a piece of writing, we can say: 'I don't really know who wrote this, what it may be about or what its value is.'

The time needed for this exercise varies, of course, according to the context. An hour and a half is enough for most situations, but it can be divided into parts of as little as ten minutes. This also depends upon the amount of stimulus text used. Here are some suggestions:

- Select a piece of your writing – an essay, diary entry, note or poem – that you wish to investigate or work further upon. You might, for example, be seeking to interpret, edit, develop or evaluate the text. Think about your purpose, but don't be too prescriptive. Rather, allow yourself to consider what you might want to do with this writing.

- Make a point of 'delivering' the writing to yourself – perhaps by putting it into an envelope to be opened at a later date.

- Leave it unopened for at least 24 hours – and preferably two or three days – to get some psychological distance from it.

- At the appointed time, open the text and choose from the following to say (aloud, I suggest):
  ◦ I wonder what this writing has to say to me
  ◦ I wonder who wrote it
  ◦ I wonder how I will feel when I read it
  ◦ I wonder what I will think about it
  ◦ I wonder what I will do with it.

- Now read, reminding yourself that you do not 'know' the author.

- After the first reading, take a blank sheet and write a question – e.g. 'What is this about?'

- Allocate about five minutes for freewriting in response. Take your pen and just write whatever comes to mind with no censorship or correction. If your mind is blank, simply write the question – again and again – until new ideas arrive. No stopping! No correcting! No conscious thinking!

- Once you have finished, go back to the text and scan it again briefly.

- Repeat the freewriting process for each relevant question – reminding yourself that you are reading an unknown text by an unknown writer.

Students, colleagues and counselling clients alike have been pleased – and often surprised – to see how pertinent questions have arisen and new perspectives opened up. For example:

- For a counselling client, writing a long-delayed letter to his father, it helped him to see through the parent's eyes in a way he had not previously been able to do.

- For a student on a degree course in criminal justice, it inspired her to begin comparing her writing with that of journal articles and professional reports for the first time; to hone her style and to earn better grades.

- For a lecturer who tried this recently, it helped him restructure some key ideas more clearly, and to communicate them better to his students.

This exercise is a journey of investigation where the reader/writer (whoever we may be) is gently encouraged to approach writing as, at least in part, unknown. For me it also encourages deeper journeying: towards allowing, valuing and welcoming the unknown, and acknowledging its constant presence in our lives.

Memory Books   *Angie Butler*

> I came from a large family. There was mother, father, myself and
> three more sisters and three brothers, also my two aunts and two
> uncles living with us as well. My aunts and uncles were all blind.
> We lived in a small cottage with two bedrooms, a small sitting
> room, a medium sized kitchen and small back kitchen. There
> wasn't a bathroom and the toilet was outside. With only one
> toilet it was sometimes very chaotic. Someone was always
> waiting for someone else to come out so that they could go. It
> wasn't very nice when it was really windy and wet going outside
> to use the toilet especially when it was dark but we were used to
> it. The only water supply came from a tap outside the back door.
> We were lucky as years before water came from a pump in the
> farmyard. To wash the dishes after meals two large enamel bowls
> were used, one for washing and one for draining the dishes.
> Even though they were blind my aunties helped out each day
> when I was small. They also helped peel some of the vegetables
> for mother. Living like this we never had any room of our own
> like today and we all had to share a bed with someone else,
> sometimes even three to a bed…

And so the story unfolded, better than any history book, a story of real life
that had only been told in snippets before, and probably only to the close
family who had heard or lived the stories anyway. Those of us who heard
the story for the first time were gripped. That such an extraordinary life
story was written so easily. And suddenly the teller was able to feel proud of
her life and the amazing tales she could tell. I was working on a project
with Family Learning, a part of adult education. It was based in a
school whose head teacher was keen to involve grandparents and great-
grandparents in the children's learning. At each of the 13 sessions (we had
to extend the time, as the adults felt they wanted to carry on), six adults
gathered in a room in the school, anxious to share their past with their
grandchildren and great-grandchildren.

   The children drew pictures for the Memory Books, learnt to knit,
helped cook and eat potato cakes and enjoyed riding around in a cart, a
dilly, that one of the great-grandparents made for the children. The
sessions ended with a celebration assembly at the end of the spring term
when the adults shared some of their memories with the whole school, and
a recording session on local radio in July. It didn't set out to be any more
than a sharing of their grandparents' lives with the children but the value to

the adults became apparent by their comments, involvement and effort. The chance to write about their lives, each extraordinary in its own way. To be able to have in the family a real-life account that could be passed down to generations to come.

I valued my small part in encouraging them to write in their own ways and in their own voices. One gentleman wrote as if his five-year-old great-grandchild was telling his story. It made it more special to him and gave him a bond with the five-year-old, who he might not see grow up. For each session I prepared a focus, a knitted dishcloth, a wicker carpet beater, a washboard or old photographs. These stirred old memories and animated conversations between the senior people. Because the sessions were held in the school which many had attended in their youth and the children were in learning mode, I felt that the seven children of varying ages listened more attentively than they might have done at home with the distraction of family and television. The sessions lasted for two hours with half an hour without the children at the beginning and end of each session. These became an important time for the adults to share what they had been able to do at home and to share the many photographs of the village and their lives in the past.

The time with the children was spent explaining their lifestyles, cooking and eating or drawing pictures to go with the texts the adults had written. Listening to the comments of the older generation at the end of the project it was so very obvious that they had enjoyed the chance to write their stories which their families would value more and more in the years to come: a chance that would not have occurred naturally. I was privileged to have been part of such a project. One gentleman said he would never stop writing, he had loved every minute and each new memory written down stirred another memory to be written down the next day. The books varied tremendously: some handwritten, some typed by willing family members and some so comprehensive as to become time capsules in their own right with pockets full of cuttings, school reports and precious memories from outings of the past. These were given a real worth when added to the Memory Book, instead of lying at the bottom of a drawer. I think such a project could be an important part of every school's history curriculum and help many senior people feel that their lives and memories are treasures that have shaped their children's future.

One-to-One Creative Writing Therapy Sessions   *Jo Monks*

My unusual situation was this: I had a friend who was in desperate need of help and unable to find a suitable therapist. She finally came to me, not a professional therapist but a creative writing/arts practitioner. My initial reaction to helping a close friend in this way rang loud alarm bells. Boundaries were a significant concern. My immediate reaction was to dismiss the idea as unmanageable and unethical, especially since she was in such emotional need. Yet I wanted to help a close friend and was concerned by the state of her mental, emotional and physical health, particularly as she had a debilitating stomach condition.

I agreed to give regular one-hour healing arts sessions, using creative writing, drama and art, and to continue until we both agreed that it was time to stop. It was an interesting challenge for me since I had never worked on a one-to-one basis before. My background is in working with vulnerable groups of adults within a therapeutic context using drama and creative writing. What I found in these one-to-one sessions was that there were many similarities with both the process and results of working in a group setting.

The sessions took place around a table in my flat. This may not have been the ideal location, yet it was a private quiet space and I had a variety of invaluable resources at hand to improvise with if needed. These included an array of percussion instruments, costumes, masks, crayons, coloured paper, wigs, bean-bags, glue, glitter and props of various kinds. In almost every session I used some or all of these.

I planned each session and because I saw my friend Jabeen on a regular basis I became aware of what she needed and the emotions she was going through. I was flexible in my approach, and usually veered away from my plan according to what transpired, and what I perceived Jabeen needed to express at the time. I believe now that working with a close friend was in fact an asset. Jabeen had been struggling for a long time to find friends or professionals who could understand her feelings. I gained a greater understanding of her thoughts and feelings which inevitably helped us in our own friendship. It was also easier to listen and to hear her within a professional context than casually as friends. Significantly she found that artistic expression through creative writing and drama enabled her to express herself more fully than through the limitations of verbal expression. The sessions brought transformation and healing for both of us.

Jabeen had done very little creative writing, but had written some poetry and attempted to share her writing with others. However, she found this difficult as she tended to write in the first person and expressed herself in a very direct way, not viewing this as 'creative'. She consequently felt exposed and limited in how deeply she was able to express herself when sharing with others. With this in mind I intended to present very simple writing exercises in the sessions, but also to find ways in which Jabeen could distance herself from her emotions through imaginative writing.

In Session Six, 'My Ideal World', I asked Jabeen to close her eyes and visualise her ideal world, imagining its colours, sights, sounds, smells and whether there were other beings, creatures or people in this world. After a few minutes I asked her to draw this world using crayons, chalks and coloured paper. Jabeen looked very happy doing both these. I next asked her to write a description of this world which she read out to me. She then completed the process with a vocal sound and movement to express other dimensions of her world.

I next asked her to imagine and draw a destruction or invasion taking place in this world. Jabeen looked very angry as she drew and told me her picture was of 'anger'. She also told me that she had had a stomach pain when our session began but that following her expression of 'anger' this pain reduced and she felt more energised.

Jabeen then wrote a dialogue between her and 'Anger', revealing a conflict of interests. 'Anger' wanted a totally different life to her. I asked Jabeen to visualise and draw 'Anger's ideal world. This was surprisingly similar to the first drawing but Jabeen kept mentioning the word 'real' in reference to 'Anger's world. I asked Jabeen to write a second dialogue between her and 'Anger' where they both exchange information about their different worlds. 'Anger' gave her 'Reality' which in her words 'make the nasty things seen not hidden'; Jabeen gave 'Anger' unconditional love.

Jabeen drew a picture of an integrated world where she and 'Anger' live together. In this drawing 'Anger' emerged as the attacker in the form of storms. I asked if there was anything she was not happy with in this new world and she mentioned the adverse weather conditions. Discussing this further, she concluded that bad weather is only temporary and its contrast is needed in order to appreciate the sun. The session concluded with a vocal sound to reduce tension and to open up communication channels which made Jabeen feel stronger. I asked her to draw a final picture which she drew as a red and golden sun.

Jabeen experienced a range of different thoughts and emotions throughout the session, and ended feeling something had moved, transformed within her, and there were new insights which gave her a better understanding of herself. Most importantly, it was an opportunity for Jabeen to be heard and to express herself when often difficult emotions remain hidden, even from her own awareness, manifesting as debilitating and painful physical symptoms. Jabeen found the tools and the channel in which to express her most difficult emotions with a witness who was there to listen.

Freedom to Express *by Jabeen*

The sessions I had with Jo were exactly what I needed at the time and were truly transformative for me. The sessions sometimes felt like little rituals that helped me to express and then transform difficult emotions to energy that I could use to help move me forward in the present. The proactive and expressive nature of the sessions helped me to experience, within a safe space, how uncomfortable emotions can be used constructively. In a low state I often find it very challenging to express my feelings verbally so the range of creative mediums Jo had command of really helped. For the first time in my life I felt that I really had the opportunity to express my feelings in whatever form worked for me in a non judgemental space. At the end of each session I felt like I had been able to work through feelings and blocks and receive deep insights.

As a result of the success of these sessions we now collaborate offering healing and arts sessions.

The Journey of Life: A Workshop with Teenage Cancer Patients   *Gillie Bolton*

The activity therapist canvassed the ward: 'Who'd like to do some writing today? It's great fun; you'll enjoy it. Yes I do think you're well enough. You can always come back to bed if you've had enough after a few minutes – just give it a try.'

This is a teenage cancer unit. It's small and intimate, and the nurses don't wear uniforms. Many photographs adorn the walls: bald amputated patients in wheelchairs or on crutches, a celebrity's arm draped around each. Pop stars and sporting celebrities are generous to these suffering young people. A pool table takes up most of the space between the beds, and a huge plasma television dominates the day room. We clear away the habitual litter of games and magazines from the day room's huge comfy sofas, and ransack the activity cupboard for paper and coloured pens.

These young people (aged 11–20) all have cancer; many will lose a leg, if they have not already done so; many will die. All are cared for by a dedicated team with skill and deep compassion mixed with as much humour and lightness as possible.

Here we are then, settled in the day room: five children, one from West Africa, a second-generation African-Caribbean from the inner city, two from the outer city, one from Antigua, her mum, the activity therapist and me. Who am I? I am doing research into therapeutic or personal development writing, based in a university department. I have permission from the Trust ethics committee, and the support of the senior oncologist and ward sister. We will later be asking these young writers what writing has meant to them – has it been helpful or not in any way; have they enjoyed it?

They all look at me, carefully chosen coloured felt-tips poised above plain paper reinforced by big books on laps; the bleep and hum of drip stands and the muted din of London outside, forming a chorus to the quiet expectation.

'You are going on a journey,' I tell them. 'I don't know where; you'll find out as you go along. I do know you are going on a magic carpet – a big safe one. We are going to make a list of all the things we'll need on our journey. Each one of us will make a list. We'll start with clothing. What do you think you'll need?' Everyone scribbles. This is easy; they don't need to know where they're going or what it'll be like. People of that age, especially with their experience of need, know what kind of thing is essential on a journey.

We slowly worked through all sorts of different needs we might have, from the straightforward and physical, to the psychological and spiritual. Though of course I don't express these elements that way. When we come to the latter, I ask them to think of something else they might need, something when they were on their own perhaps, something to help them be brave and to cope with whatever might happen to them on their journey.

When each element has been written, we read them to each other; this constant sharing of writing is supportive, and helps the less confident ones to feel it's fine to write ordinary things like 'socks', and 'rice and peas'. It is also a very unthreatening way for them to share areas with which some feel

more confident than others, such as the spiritual. And it breaks up the
writing time into manageable small pieces.

This particular session took about an hour and a half. In retrospect this
seems a long time for what we did, but that's because I forget just how
poorly and slow those children are. If you add on the settling of people and
drips, and the very slow ending in which they sat and looked at each other,
and then begin to chat quietly before moving back to the ward, you'd need
a couple of hours for this sort of group.

It was a good way to start writing with a patient group of whose
stamina I was unsure. Later sessions we wrote long stories; but that was
once they'd got the bit between their teeth with writing, and I felt more
confident of not giving them too much to do.

Here is Josephine's journey. I haven't told you all the elements I asked
them to list, because you can work them out from her writing. I just made it
up as I went along.

My Journey by Josephine Ackomaning

I will need:
a light green polo neck jumper
heavy black tracksuit trousers
a warm winter coat
trainers or boots
socks
And a thick snuggly pale mauve blanket
corned beef and sweetcorn sandwiches
hot and cold drinks
sweet pastries
and rice and peas
my medication
a penknife
toothbrush and toothpaste
a mobile phone so I can phone home
a walkman to play travelling funk music
or Cools whatever my mood
and a magical dog called Risky
who is brown

a cuddly size
and can talk and be invisible
Protection and guidance from God
which might be helpful or comforting
I feel it when I'm quiet
and when I'm praying
I pray quietly
Some magical medication
to prevent me getting sick
and courage which is white.
We need a white motor boat
some firewood and firelighters
tents
some rain coats
cooking pans
cutlery
some cushions and pillows
some towels
and a camera to take photos to take home

We will arrive at a tropical island with fruit and vegetables
with no one else there just me and Risky
and Risky and I will have fun.

I've also used a similar workshop with adult psychiatric in-patients. They needed far less warming up with lists of clothing and food, and dived into psychological and spiritual needs with verve and sparkle, with imagination and very great need. I wasn't able to keep copies of writings from those men (it was chance they were all men, including the member of staff who joined in). But although it was several years ago, I vividly remember their excitement and joy as they scribbled their list-poems, and read back the things which they felt they needed to succour them on their journey of life.

CHAPTER 10

Loss and Change

Edited by Kate Thompson

Throughout the life course we are constantly subject to loss and change. Change can be consciously sought and determined or thrust upon us. As the principal of a college said somewhat oxymoronically in her annual address, 'Change is here to stay'. Change is inevitably accompanied by loss; sometimes that loss is to be welcomed, sometimes it is to be struggled with and needs to be worked through. Writing can be a very helpful way of reaching a different kind of understanding of the self in all its different phases.

The contributors in this chapter write about loss and change, in different contexts and with different age groups, both invited and unexpected.

Loss of youth

Even children lose their childhood if they have disturbing or damaging experiences. Carry Gorney uses storymaking with her young client to help him recover from the effects of traumatic abuse. She joins him in the creation of narratives about the Humfylumph, a mythical creature who embodies David and his demons and helps David to recover his sense of playfulness and creativity. When working with people who cannot, for some reason, write their own words, the act of becoming their scribe creates an intimate bond which is itself a healing relationship. Carry acts as the scribe for David; in Judy Clinton's piece carers become scribes for their disabled clients.

Loss of relationships

Loss of relationships can be traumatic through bereavement or rejection but it can also be ultimately about growth. In Briony Goffin's piece her student writes about finding herself in a situation where she is stripped of all the expectations of other relationships; through the diary format she is able to relate directly to herself. Writing in this way people are often able to develop a new intimacy with the self, unmediated by other perspectives or relationships.

Unsent letters

Many clients come to therapy because of issues of loss and change which are often to do with relationships. In Dear Ray…Love Jean, Jean discovers her true feelings about her husband and his departure through writing him an unsent letter. When she reads it she is surprised by the nature of the feelings it reveals. Just as unsent letters can be used for exploring current relationships they are also powerful instruments for use in bereavement.

Just because someone dies that's no reason to stop writing them letters (Michaels 1996). Writing unsent letters to someone who has died is a way of keeping them involved in the life of the family, keeping their memory alive. It can be a way of resolving past difficulties and understanding relationships differently. Elaine was a 60-year-old woman who had cared for her mother who died. Her grief was complicated by her guilt at feeling some relief but what also emerged through her unsent letters to her mother was anger at her siblings for their lack of support for her in the role of carer. Subsequently she was able to talk to her siblings about this and developed a much closer relationship with her sister.

With present relationships writing unsent letters can provide a way of resolving current difficulties and finding a different perspective by expressing things cathartically and safely. This can be a prelude to more constructive dialogue. Unsent letters are particularly helpful for expressing anger and for revealing hidden or repressed anger which can be present in relationships and emerge insidiously.

Loss of physical health

Loss of physical health and power can be devastating for some people who develop degenerative diseases or serious debilitating conditions. Writing can be a way of reconnecting with the healthy self. In writing, as in reading, people can access different worlds and recover lost ones. In one group June, a 65-year-old woman with serious heart and lung problems, wrote a Captured Moment (Adams 1990) about reaching a Lake District summit and gained a sense of euphoria in the present through writing about a joyous experience in the past. It was a way of helping her to remember that, although her physical life was now constrained by her illness, this was not the totality of her experience and she did not have to be defined in this way. One of the group members in Judy Clinton's piece recaptures her experience of being able-bodied through writing.

In Christine Bousfield's workshop participants are guided through childhood to memories of illness and which then become narratives of healing and of understanding. She uses psychoanalytic theory as a way of interpreting and underpinning the work.

Mending the Lives of Children: The Humfylumph
Carry Gorney

This was five-year-old David's third session. He was out of control, with tantrums, having been abused two years previously: his parents were distraught because they couldn't protect him. David talked incessantly, cracked good jokes and pulled funny faces. He sat between his parents smiling like an angel, whilst they described his outbursts, voices edged with despair.

'What is he like when he has an outburst?' I asked.

They said he became 'humfy'.

'I'm like a humfylumph!' David added, excitedly.

I asked what a humfylumph looked like and he stretched his little arms out very wide.

'He takes up a lot of space,' I observed.

David nodded frowning.

'Too much space?' I enquired.

David's angry outbursts spoiled bedtimes. He longed for his story with his mum or dad but often missed it because humfylumph arrived. I asked him to describe what happened.

He jumped up shouting and ran round the room acting out the humfylumph, lurching across the floor like the hunchback of Notre Dame with terrible horns and a ferocious grimace. His narrative became very complex. David worked hard, breathlessly changing characters, a soldier fighting the angry monster to becoming the actual monster. Finally he curled up on the carpet making baby snuffles and all the time whispering the words of the story which he asked me to record:

The Humfylumph Monster: A Story with Words and Actions *by David*

The humfy would be a big monster. It would stamp and have big claws.

Humfsmonster says

'You're not my friend', to its wife. He gets a bite on the head, saying this so loud he's getting red in the face.

He needs a surprise party when he comes back from his adventure.

He's looking for some hunters that he can pick up and eat.

The hunters scream, 'There's a humfy monster.'

They get picked up by Humfy Monster and he eats the hunters.

He only

eats the bad guys

A baby person

a baby person dressed up. The real babies are in the ground so small you can't see them

They all know Humfy Monster eats people so they don't go off in the woods

Bad guy is dressed as a baby, robot dressed in clothes holds baby

Know what they are going to eat by the smell

Should be good in the story

Might know that they're not bad guys

David asked his mum to read his story out whilst he sat on his dad's knee, sucking his thumb. When she had finished, he handed it to me before leaving at the end of the session.

David and his parents were attending the Child and Adolescent Mental Health Service in Sheffield, where I work as a family therapist; part of a multidisciplinary team with a common aim to help mend the lives of children. My responsibility was to help David mould and breathe life into a new preferred story about himself.

David had drawn the story of his abuse with his body. He allowed his narrative to inhabit his physical being just as his unresolved anger had inhabited his everyday world. His fear had metamorphosed into anger; the drama mirrored the frightening abuse and David conquered it, witnessed by adults. Witnessing David's journey through the difficulties seemed an essential part of his healing. David understood his parents respected and believed his portrayal of the emotional trauma which had been his experience.

He drew on ever-changing thoughts, images and metaphors to feed his imagination. The stories were laid out as puzzles of apparently disconnected ideas. He used words as reflections of his internal landscape which became part of his external landscape during our sessions. I wrote alongside him, capturing moments to preserve this child's magic. If David could recognise his own creative qualities, he could believe in his own capacity to heal himself. He communicated metaphorically. Eventually the story would unfold.

> By putting into words I can make it whole; this way it has lost the power to hurt me. (Virginia Woolf 1978, p.72)

David was able to put the horrors and fears surrounding his traumatic experience into drama and actions, giving me the role of ghost writer to record his story.

With a child's ability to leap into the surreal world of magic and monsters he was able to create the humfylumph. This monstrous creature was no longer a secret in the deep recesses of David's mind. As soon as the monster had been externalised, David would no longer dig a deep hole within himself. He was able to find form for the monster and place it outside, amongst those he trusted. It would become a diluted part of everyone's experience and eventually dissolve into the ether.

To summarise, this is what happened:

- We turned the abuse into a humfylumph monster.

- We created space for David to act out the complex story.

- We seized the moment David said 'I'm like a humfylumph monster' as the cue to create something outside David himself, which could be conquered.

- When David saw his story on paper he understood he was no longer fighting alone, the adults could take over.

- David delivered his frightening narrative with humour and dramatic intensity.

- We all collaborated to invent a character which David could use to communicate his innermost fears.

- When David started acting out his narrative there was no further need for me to ask questions, I simply needed to record his performance.

- David's parents gave us the words and the cues to build this drama.

- I wrote because David liked words and used them eloquently.

- He told us the story when he was ready, in Session Three.

- I made no effort to change or explain what he acted/wrote. It belonged to him.

Finally David drew a picture of himself very wobbly on stilts.

> It's hard to be big and balance...you need help from your Mum and Dad.

Writing in Spite of Physical Barriers   *Judy Clinton*

I have been facilitating writing groups for some years now, in the interests of personal and spiritual awareness and growth. I believe profoundly in the power of writing spontaneously, and the sharing of those writings, to reveal, heal and inspire. My interest has never been in end results, but in the process of creation and expression. My experience has taught me that when a group of people come together in an open way, in a safe space, 'things happen' through the writing and sharing process.

I ran a series of sessions, funded by the charity Scope, for physically disabled people in a local day centre. This client group was new to me. It was a huge challenge for me, with remarkable results.

When I arrived for the first session I discovered that those who had been prepared to engage with the process had the most complex set of practical disabilities and range of writing experience that I could possibly have imagined. I had two ladies with visual impairments – one young woman had been completely blind since birth; the other, a lady in her seventies, had macular degeneration and could only see out of one small part of one eye. A Caribbean lady had advanced multiple sclerosis and struggled to find speech; she was also wheelchair bound and unable to write. A young woman with cerebral palsy, also wheelchair bound, had no speech and communicated through a series of squeals, cries and loud bursts of laughter. One older lady had severe dyslexia and described herself as having 'sleepy brain'. Two ladies had suffered severe strokes and were wrestling with a variety of coordination problems of body and mind. Another lady, also with multiple sclerosis, had more minor practical difficulties with getting words onto paper.

However, it was quite amazing what we did manage to achieve. Those people in the group who could not write for themselves had carers from the day centre, who knew them well, as their scribes. The young blind lady used a Braille typewriter, whilst those who could write did their best to do so. I was deeply moved to see how carers and service users worked together to put down in words on a page that which the service user struggled to express. In the case of the young woman with cerebral palsy, the carer would write what she believed the young woman would say and then read it back to her – if the young woman was in agreement with it she would smile and laugh, at other times showing in no uncertain terms that her scribe had got it wrong. In this way, together, they painstakingly worked to express what the body-locked young woman wanted to say. A similar process went on with the lady with advanced multiple sclerosis. It was rather like working with three-legged racers at times; carers wrote and listened, and service users worked to say what burned within them.

A range of subjects was dealt with in an entirely spontaneous manner: I asked them to write down the first thing that came into their heads in response to a given subject, and then to write the next thing that occurred to them, going on a kind of adventure trail within their own thoughts and feelings. This method worked extremely well as it did not rely on planning and literary skill, which many would have found beyond them. I used a variety of stimuli, the most powerful being the use of a tape of the sounds of the sea. The lady with multiple sclerosis said with a beaming smile, after she had heard her piece read out to the group, 'I wasn't just remembering that, I was doing it.'

> I was walking in a quiet stream through stones in the water. The wind was blowing, the sun was shining. Seen a puddle. I was throwing a stone in the water, the wind was blowing in my face. I was looking forward, I was walking towards the beach. The wind was blowing. I picked up a few stones and threw them in the water, even though the sun was shining, I was throwing stones in a puddle. The seagull was making a noise above my head while I was throwing stones in the water, because the wind

was blowing toward me, I was throwing a stone. I was skipping along on the beach, that was what I was doing. I was feeling happy with myself, while the wind was blowing.

For the short period of time during which she was writing this she was able-bodied again. It was a precious time for us all. Strong emotions of sorrow, frustration, happiness, anger, and everything in between, found expression within that group during the course.

Part of my remit from Scope was to ask people to write about their disabilities, to give them an opportunity to express how it was for them to be disabled people in our society. Those writings were deeply moving and although they were at times sad and full of pain there was also a great deal of laughter and philosophical insight that was shared. Service users said how good it had been to share in this way and to learn about each other's problems and ways of dealing with them. One lady wrote about the loss of several years of her life as a result of the misdiagnosis of her condition. She told me afterwards that she had never written of those feelings before, nor shared them with anybody else, and how healing this had been.

Although the group was a very verbal one, and a higher proportion of time was spent in sharing writings and discussing what came out of them than actually writing, the writing process was very important. This was the time during which people turned inwards and expressed creatively what was present within them at that point in time. For people who are so severely limited in how they can operate in the world, this is a marvellously satisfying and liberating thing to do. At the end of the course I compiled a booklet of members' writings and gave each person a copy to keep. The pleasure of seeing their names in print, and of having a record of what had been shared within the group, was a delight to see. My belief that 'things happen' when people come together to write in this way has been fully validated by this experience.

Thanks to *Writer's Forum*. A version of this piece appeared in October 2005.

Exploring Childhood: Lacan and Kristeva

Christine Bousfield

This was a workshop at the Lapidus conference, April 2004. Twenty-one people attended, several experienced writers amongst them used to working in poetry and health care. 'Exploring childhood' was clearly relevant to this year's conference theme 'Writing the Life Journey' and to psychoanalytic approaches in general. My comments here reflect my interests in mother–child relationships, ambivalence, unconscious repetition between generations, physical illness and the salutary effects of working through all these in writing.

I have developed this technique through practice on myself, on MA literature and MA psychoanalysis students at Leeds Metropolitan University, at Harrogate Hospital with child and adult insulin-dependent diabetics, and with Mind in Leeds.

We began at the level of 'free association' or 'freewriting' with the trigger words 'Mother' or 'Father' or 'Sister' or 'Brother'. Then we moved to the second stimulus, 'a childhood illness' recalled again in free associative writing. Participants were asked to rework an extract from the morning's writing into a draft poem, thinking of a sculptor working on raw stone (the associations) but always allowing the pulse, the music and the play on words, what we might call the implicit *desire* of the poem, to take precedence.

One or two participants found writing about significant others, childhood experience and illness difficult; most said the workshop was sometimes disturbing but well handled and there were particular comments about the fruitfulness of transferring associations from one scenario to another (poetically speaking).

Even before we began writing, one person became 'inexplicably full of tears' (her words). Paradoxically, this acted as a stimulus for the group so that, in the poetry that followed, silence, lack and absence occurred both in poetic form and as a theme. In a sense the group was 'put in process' through this 'absent poem'.

Another participant could not write anything but the word 'No' and in the feedback wrote that the workshop was too heavy for a conference. However, she finally sent me a poem and thanked me for enabling it.

My justification here is that some writers, I feel, are ready to confront difficult issues/memories: there is, after all, plenty of scope for evasive writing, in any case carrying hidden symptoms, silences, metaphors and displacements.

Kate Evans evoked the repetition between generations in her poem 'A Mother's Love':

> Hers was a desperate attempt
> not to do what her mother had done.
> Instead of chaos, she would have calm.
> Instead of venom she would have only minted words.

Don't we eat mint to cover up bad breath? Are there implications of bad breath, or of bad faith here? We also think of coins, symbolic currency, as 'minted' and capable of legitimate exchange beyond 'venom'. Indeed the poet refers ironically to economics:

> two would have done just fine
> a boy and a girl,
> in terms of population and environmental balance –
> the right replacement value

Here the third child identifies with a maternal grandmother consciously rejected by her mother. Many of us have been there!

> she…resents her gift
> tosses it back
> into her startled face
>
> turns…minted words to venom.

Here there is a complete reversal of her mother's reported habits but clearly repetition in her opposition to the maternal figure.

Another poet, C, associates winter with home/mother and

> A time of ungrowing,
> unravelling, time inside

There are evocations of a joyless Christmas when the subject is imprisoned in stillness:

> On every wide red window sill
> My mother set still life: holly, lemons
> candles pale and unlit. Still lives. Outside
> some star that I should have been following
> passed by, on the other side.

Here there are biblical associations in the missed star and abandonment when all but the Samaritan 'passed by, on the other side'.

C compares herself to a white hyacinth:

> A pale bulb, rooted in dark,
> brought out too soon, forced
> to flower.

Here there is ambivalence about separation, the longing to leave, to follow desire together with complaints about abandonment. Strangely, the subject's daughters, the next generation, appear to escape this ambivalence:

> in lush unweeded summer
> I watch closely my daughters;
> their curves of perfect fitting skin
> their unstilled growing limbs
> their lightness, flowering.

This is a complex poem, with many quotations and allusions. The 'unweeded garden' for Hamlet is an image of lust (particularly women's): here it is reconceived as freedom and lushness.

Several participants, not surprisingly, worked through a period of illness. Kate Thompson, for instance, strikingly articulates her desire to move upwards and outwards from the abjection of her 'iron bed' through the 'ward window pane' to the

> Aeroplane an ant across the sky
> Boat an ant across the water
> Lincolnshire the thin strip of horizon.

She effectively re-symbolises recovering from a brain tumour in terms of the building of the Humber Bridge, compared to the stitching/bandaging of her 'shaven skull':

> They are building the Humber Bridge,
> Delicate lines slicing the plane of river-sea and sky
> Helicopter drivelling the final section into place
>
> Neatly closing the central gap, surprising,
> I thought a bridge goes from the near bank to the far
> But no, completion grows from each end reaching out to
> the other

Here there is the movement from the abjection of a gap/wound in the head into something more culturally recognised and bearable, the bridge as symbolic of closure and healing.

Graham Hartill symbolises home/garden and the outside/beyond in very ambivalent fashion, in terms of over-sweetness and monstrosity, imprisonment and freedom, terror and safety:

> The garden is walled...
> But everything is in the garden
> The garden is full of lions
> The garden is perfumed with sugar

Here there is an allusion to the biblical line 'from the strong come forth sweetness' famously used by Tate & Lyle on their treacle tins. Of course, 'sugar' is often associated with 'mother', 'home' and love.

Later the poet asks whether the 'head' is monstrous or has a human face, and tries to decide if the monster is *outside* or *inside* the garden. This tallies very much with Freud's theory of the uncanny as 'something hidden and dangerous...[which] develop[s] so that "heimlich" [literally "homely"] comes to have the meaning usually ascribed to "unheimlich" ["uncanny"]' (Freud 1985, p.346) which he also connects with the mother:

> It has to be a head
> It has to have a head
> The head is everything
> The head is safety [of recognition]

Notice the repeated return to the same place yet with developing articulation and extension. Graham, in another piece written to his mother, thanks her for reading to him when constantly ill as a child (she provides symbolic resources, sublimation, for him in his sickness/abjection). He recognises he is part of her 'fantasy about good books that I was to fulfil' yet claims freedom from the mother's desire through the development of his own imagination, not 'for you. Beyond you.' There he is undoing the debt to his mother and establishing separation, if a little abruptly and enviously! Later he uses the word, 'gestation': pregnancy is often claimed by (male) poets and artists. Perhaps this ending could also be a more positive introjection of the mother, bringing about identity transformation.

During this workshop, I presented myself explicitly as a fellow traveller into the unconscious with all my human issues and frailties. However, I tried to listen and make comments more impersonally from a linguistic point of view, in order to encourage more resonance. I also focused on the poetry more as an articulation of what is or has been unspeakable, not simply for the poet/speaker but for all subjects founding themselves on a language in transformation, poetic language.

Thanks here to C, Kate Evans, Kate Thompson and Graham Hartill for allowing me to discuss their poems.

Dear Ray...Love Jean   *Kate Thompson*

Unsent Letters is one of the most versatile of therapeutic writing techniques; it can be used with individuals or groups, in isolation or in workshops. There is a familiarity in writing letters which people find comforting; it is a known task with an understood purpose.

It is a technique that is suitable for people who know they have strong emotion to express and want to vent it safely in the search for catharsis and also for people who are unaware of their emotions; it can facilitate the expression of unacknowledged feeling. I have used it frequently when there are issues of loss – in grief work writing letters to the deceased loved one can be a useful part of the healing process.

This is the story of one woman who was referred by her GP to the practice counsellor because of, in the euphemistic words characteristic of some GP referrals, 'relationship problem' and 'stress' – her husband had left the family home saying that he needed some space but, it later emerged, he had moved in with another (younger) woman, leaving Jean with three children and a mountain of debt he had incurred, mostly in her name.

The setting: a nurse's room in a GP practice, littered with the accoutrements of medicine: jars, bottles, old-fashioned scales, a medicine fridge, faded anatomical posters. We sit on hard, moulded chairs angled towards each other. It is our third meeting. In our first meeting we discussed the possibility of using writing as part of our work; Jean recalled keeping a diary as a teenager but said she hadn't written since. In the second session she is calm but a bit bewildered, like a lost child. She said she'd always loved him and couldn't understand why he had left her. She still hoped he would return to them but he was not answering her calls, although he would let himself into the house unannounced to see the children. He was still living with the other woman.

I sensed something else beneath the childlike presentation, something denied.

I suggested that Jean go and write a letter to her husband, this man who had left her with three children and a mountain of debt, this man who she said she wanted to return to her. Before she started writing she had to promise herself two things:

1. that she would never send the letter

2. that she would allow herself to write whatever came into her mind. Her writing was free to be uncensored – all the things she would say to him, all the things she had been telling me, all the questions (*Why? Why? Why?*) that were unanswered. She could say what she really thought and express what she really felt.

When we meet for the third time she looks embarrassed, her mouth offers a little smile but her eyes, looking up from under her fringe, contain a new expression of defiance. She meets my look and pulls some sheets of lined paper out from her shiny handbag.

'I've done it, like you said. Only it wasn't what I thought. At first it was hard, real hard. I didn't know how to begin. But when I started – I didn't want to stop, it all came out. It's not like me, not me at all. Can I read it to you?'

As she begins to read her voice is tremulous, timid, and almost apologetic as she had been in many of our conversations so far.

> Dear Ray
>
> I don't know why I'm writing to you. My counsellor suggested it, I'm having counselling because of what's happened. I wish you'd talk to me. I'm writing to you because you are not answering my calls, I don't know why you won't talk to me. Billy wants to know why you won't talk to him – he's only 11, what's he done?
>
> Why can't we just talk? I want to understand... I don't understand.
>
> When we met I was 17 and I thought the world of you. You were so big and strong – a bit too strong sometimes but I knew you loved me.

But as she continues her voice becomes stronger.

> When you left you said you wanted some space, I believed you. Of course I know it's hard with the kids, noise, no money – it's hard for me too. Actually it is hard for me, yes, it is. Sometimes I would have liked to go out, dance like we used to, but you can't with three, can you? You can't expect to. I couldn't but you

> didn't think of that – you went out when you wanted, or taking
> out a loan in my name I never saw. Why did you do that?

A new voice begins to emerge, louder, more expressive, carrying more
emotion, not so crushed by life, some energy and expression in her tone.

The letter begins with the plaintive, pleading tone of the bewildered
child but metamorphoses through injured complaint to indignation and
invective. She becomes angry and this new expression of emotion startles
us both with its vehemence.

> Well Ray, I don't understand, and perhaps you can't explain,
> won't more like I ask WHY? WHY? WHY? But it's just you, you
> you always were selfish, didn't think of anyone else. SELFISH.
> SELFISH MAN.
>
> Must go
>
> Love, Jean

It is the first time she has given vent to these feelings; indeed until she wrote
the letter she had been unable to recognise or acknowledge her anger.
When she finished reading her eyes shone and her breathing was quicker –
gone was the timid, depressed figure of earlier.

'What do you notice when you read this out loud? What do you hear?'

'Two things – I was always afraid of him and now I am angry with him.
The bastard. Funny that, I'm not an angry sort of person.' And she was no
longer embarrassed by feeling.

In a workshop, or as self-guided writing, I ask people to give themselves this kind of feedback in writing. This allows them to reflect upon
their spontaneous writing and to recognise some of the underlying feelings
which so often emerge in writing.

Unsent Letters are always that – unsent. They may provide the first
draft of a letter that is sent but the original is kept or destroyed. In this case
the writer tore her letter into tiny pieces and flushed it down the lavatory.
Repressing her anger had contributed to her depression, writing the letter
had released it.

Writing as Evolution   *Briony Goffin*

On Thursday mornings, eight individuals trickle out of the folds in the
landscape and make their way to the Landmark Shed. This is an old farm
building, now half artist studio, half 'writing room', on the side of a hill in
rural Somerset. It is full of plants and speckled mirrors, has paint-splashed

walls and needs four portable radiators to keep it warm. In the midst of the elements, this group is vibrant and familiar. In 2003 they had each responded to an advert for one of my beginners' creative writing courses. Now, nearly three years on, they continue to come together to experience themselves as multifaceted beings who are rich with imagery and ideas, to transcend their everyday roles as parent, partner, child, employer, employee and become – become whatever!

The first half of their session is usually shaped around some free-writing, prompted by a topic or stimulus that I bring to the group. On the last Thursday of this November, I offered them the choice of either writing from the perspective of someone hiding or writing from the perspective of someone who is running away. I asked them to express whatever was intuitively aroused by either of these notions, attending in particular to sensation and feeling. I encouraged them to resist the inclination towards explanation but rather to immerse themselves in the imagery. I offered them no suggestions or examples – I didn't define whether running away or hiding should be a positive or negative event, or whether it could be a literal or metaphorical exploration. The action of hiding or running away makes evolutionary sense in response to conditions of stress, loss and change. Whichever direction they took, the chosen event was likely to demonstrate the human condition in all its rawness, asking of writing that it pulsate with intense and personal drama. It felt important that my role was one of containing, rather than guiding, to see (and trust in) what emerged organically.

In recent weeks, these conditions seemed to facilitate a curious and strangely gratifying phenomenon, in which words and ideas began to echo one another across the group. Individuals were finding that the last line of their work was actually the title of the work belonging to the individual opposite, or the writing they had chosen to share from home had utterly tuned into the theme I had chosen for the session. Whether this is sublime synchronicity or an outcome of multi-levelled communication is a juicy question yet to be answered.

Today it became apparent that the themes of concealment and escape were to resonate throughout everything. The second half of the session is usually characterised by one group member sharing a piece of work developed at home. The rest of the group is then invited to respond to the ideas, imagery and language and I, in the meantime, record everything, aiming to capture the spirit of this exchange, to provide the writer with a permanent account of all the feedback before its subtle flavours dissipate. This week it was Bridget's turn. As her story unfolded, it soon became clear that she, too, had unwittingly produced something that linked up all the conceptual threads of the session, binding it into something that was to become cohesive and distinct. Her piece traced a woman's experience of running away to Cornwall over Christmas time.

Diary Extracts by Bridget

> I don't know how it feels to be alone, just me, it feels odd looking at everyone else in couples or families eating fish and chips, I drink hot chocolate. I quite like being just me, not daughter, mother, wife, lover. I do exist on my own, that's a surprise… I have brought a sketchbook with me, I'm going to keep a visual diary as well if I can, I need to have evidence that I do exist on my own… I can feel people looking at me and wondering what I am scribbling to myself. I will pretend this is normal for me, I can imagine I was a free spirit, and it is the most normal thing in the world for me to do, to be drawing and writing in the view of others. In fact I can be who I want to be, they don't know who I am, I don't know who I am… I've achieved something today, the words I wrote, the drawings I produced are mine, separate from anyone else. No one else can touch these things, spoil them. They are me.

At the end of her reading, the group was bursting to ask questions and respond with more of their own 'running-away' fantasies. One member said, 'What makes this writing irresistible is that you make the fantasy into reality, you take a primal human instinct and follow it through to fruition, answering some of our "what ifs" on the way.' In this transition, Bridget had shifted an experience of loss, loss of identity under the expectation of her roles, to one of evolution and gain. It was suggested that whether Bridget chose to pursue this writing as a piece of fiction or non-fiction, the idea of microscopically examining the human condition when estranged from familiar surroundings, distractions, relationships and responsibilities, to document the highs and lows and all the other notes in between, was deeply tantalising. It was particularly felt that the diary-entry format, the use of present tense and the sense of white paper as the space on which to 'work' one's self out combined to create an appealing atmosphere of intimacy and authenticity. It was an honour to be privy to this woman's interior world as she stood on the threshold of newly discovering, or redefining, her needs and vulnerabilities, her drives and desires against this 'rough' Cornish seascape at Christmas. The writing process was shown to be a dynamic tool with which to explore 'the self' in relation to a real physical and virtual emotional world. The page was like a mirror and the act of writing was like the breath that steams it up. The words were evidence of a life, vital and stirred up.

What was satisfying to me, so much so that I had to suppress my excitement like a proud creative writing mother, was that writing was perceived as a constantly available resource, not just something 'special' to Thursday mornings, or to our quirky Landmark Shed. In the face of loss and change, writing could pay heed to those faint internal voices, enabling them to be brought to the surface, as a means of making contact with oneself – maybe even the group. This is the opposite of estrangement. What was a session initially characterised by themes of hiding and running away came to be about revelation and arrival.

CHAPTER 11

Conclusion: Writing Works

Gillie Bolton, Victoria Field and Kate Thompson

Having reached the end of this book the value of writing as a tool for personal healing and growth has, we feel, been amply demonstrated. In conclusion, the three editors offer their own personal metaphors for the importance of this work. Writing for self-illumination and support can be a way of life, not just for times of despair or elation. If we are to be able to support and inspire others, writer facilitators, therapists or tutors must also write for themselves. Our own writing underpins and underscores all the work we do with others. Whatever form this writing may take, it is the process of doing it which is so vital.

Take Care by *Gillie Bolton*

You are about to enter a danger zone
Wear protective clothing around your heart
Take off your shoes

Writing can seriously damage your sadness
Writing can seriously damage your nightmares
You are in danger of achieving your dreams

Once started you won't be able to stop
Nor will you want to
And others might catch it too

You are in serious danger of learning you're alive
You are in serious danger of laughing out loud
You are in serious danger of loving yourself

If it gets in your eyes, consult your loved ones

If it gets in your mind, cancel your therapist

If it gets in your heart, hold on tight

The Woodcutter's Daughter by Kate Thompson

The poet Mary Oliver once said that when she goes for a walk she leaves pencils for people to find.

Once upon a time a woodcutter and his wife lived with their daughter in a cottage on the edge of the great forest which climbed up the mountain. The villagers lived in fear of the forest where wolves and other wild creatures roamed whose howls could be heard when darkness fell. This was used as a warning to the children of the village to persuade them of the wisdom of good behaviour and of not straying beyond the edge of the village. However, from time to time a child, overcome by curiosity or in over-zealous pursuit of a game, would disappear into the forest never to be seen again. The villagers could hear the cries of the lost children carried out of the forest on the wind and the whole village mourned.

Sometimes the woodcutter would take his daughter into the forest with him when he worked and she would play safely near him looking at the wild creatures or gathering the berries and wild flowers which grew on the forest floor.

'Never wander where you cannot hear the sound of your father's axe, child, or you may never find yourself again,' her mother warned her.

One day she was playing in a clearing, her father's axe tap-tapping in the trees nearby. A chipmunk sat on a log nibbling a stem of grass and watched her with its wise bright eyes. It ran a little distance away from her and then looked back at her until she approached, at which point it scampered further on. She continued to follow it in this way, drawn on by the wise, bright eyes, until she could hardly hear her father's axe. Girl and chipmunk were straying from the clearing into the forest itself where the trees grew closer together and daylight hardly penetrated the forest canopy at all. Their eyes began to be accustomed to the gloom and the girl could just make out silhouette of tree and bush. There were strange sounds around them, sounds of animals which did not sound benevolent but which rather howled and moaned deeper in the darkness. Then she heard a different sound, a child's plaintive cry, and could not tell whether it was her own voice or another's.

Then she knew if she went any further she could not be sure of finding her way home and perhaps would not see her mother and father or her home again but would be benighted in the forest, prey to the wild creatures that she sensed were waiting for her. Her heart grew cold with fear and she felt the inhospitable world around her; she wanted to turn and run back to the brightness of the clearing and the sound of her father's axe. But she found she could not, her feet would not obey her, she felt cold and alone. Then the chipmunk, its wise bright eyes shining in the gloom, regarded her impatiently and then turned its eyes on something in the tree. The chipmunk was looking at a thick pencil which was just within the girl's reach. She plucked it from the tree in which it rested and at that moment a broad leaf fell to the ground, its pale underside uppermost. She picked up the leaf and found that the pencil made clear marks as if the leaf were made of the finest parchment. With confident hand she wrote her name and the date and placed the leaf where the pencil had nestled; it glowed softly in the dark. Tucking the pencil in her pocket she set off after the chipmunk with renewed purpose.

The way grew darker, the undergrowth thicker and the sounds of the forest louder as they climbed steeply. From time to time the chipmunk stopped to wait for her, for it was more adept than she at movement through the thicket. When she caught up and paused she found that a leaf would fall to the ground. Each time this happened she wrote her name and the date and a few words about their journey and hung it on a tree. Each time she did this her fear diminished further.

They penetrated deeper and steeper into the heart of the forest and the wild noises around them kept them company but never approached close enough to do them harm. Eventually the trees parted and they found themselves in a clearing high up on the mountain side. They could look down and see the village far below beyond the edge of the dark forest, the village with the little white houses and the tiny figures moving between. The forest behind them was no longer entirely dark, for their path was now made visible by soft glow of the fluttering leaves on which the woodcutter's daughter had written. Huddled at the edge of the clearing the girl saw her playmates who had disappeared from the village; they were just as they were when she had last seen them as if they had stopped growing the moment they left the safety of their home. The chipmunk gave her one last look and scampered away into the forest.

The woodcutter's daughter spoke to the other children and together they began their descent. Following the leaves on which she had written, they made their way through the forest together. One by one the other children found thick pencils in the trees just within their reach and were able to write their names on leaves like finest parchment. As they did this they began to grow again until, when they emerged from the forest at the foot of the mountain and found their parents waiting for them, they inhabited once more their proper ages. Each child could look up at the mountain and trace their journey home by the leaves glowing softly against the dark foliage of the wild forest. That night there was much rejoicing in the village and the howling wolves now sounded a long way away.

Words *by Victoria Field*

after Anne Sexton

Some words fly to Ararat
soft, white and singular

Others emerge suddenly from the conjuror's cape
I'm fearful of him and his wands and witchery

My words are as quiet as toes in a shoe
and hidden like the nothing worn beneath a summer dress

My words want to fill your wellingtons with the thrill
of waves from the oceans

but they are unsteady, born too soon
and knot in my fingers like failed knitting

The poet said, 'be careful of words'
How I know what she meant –

they trap my blood to make black poppies on snow –
they love me, they love me not. (Field 2004b, p.84)

Twenty Doctors Visit an Enchanted Abbey: A Story for Children
by Gillie Bolton

The doctors weren't wearing their white coats or their steth-oscopes. They had no bags with needle and pills, bandages and sphygmomanometers. There were no couches to lie on here, no desks with computers and prescriptions. These doctors looked like anyone else: mums and dads, granddads and aunties.

But there was a difference. All these people had papers and pens. Some looked quite nervous when they arrived. They sat in groups around round tables. Except for one. She had a small bell which sounded soft, but its music sang into every ear. She was there to help these doctors to look at their ordinary old world with different eyes and ears. She wanted them to look more closely at things and people – like exactly what colour lollipop the little girl who came to the surgery was licking; what did it smell like and what did her laugh sound like.

At the very beginning the doctors looked a bit worriedly at the lady with the enchanted bell. They felt just a little anxious that the spell might not work for them. Within ten minutes, however, their pens had turned into magic wands and their paper into magic carpets. They'd forgotten exactly where they were sitting because bright memories were flowing onto the page. Well, they weren't all happy – some of the stories and poems were sad or troubled. But they were still glad they'd written them, and that they'd shared them.

These doctors, you see, all read their stories and their poems to each other. And they cried and they laughed together. And they talked about how it had felt, and how it might've been different.

And in the evening they sang songs to each other, and read poems and stories written by other people, listening spellbound, just like to bedtime stories.

By home time at the end of the weekend, the big room was filled with far more than the 20 doctors and the bell lady. There were all the children and all the grown-ups they had written and talked about, as well as the real people. The room, with its enormous Abbey window, was warm with all the voices and thoughts and memories which had been shared.

The 20 doctors all went away, and went back to their poorly patients with enchanted spectacles, hearing aids and gloves to help them see, hear and touch right through to the middle of things. And they took with them more magic carpet paper – scarlet and pink, blue and yellow, green and turquoise – to create more writing to spellbind more doctors with word-pictures of how things are, how they might be, and how they could possibly be if everything were as wonderful as possible in medicine.

Why Writing? by *Victoria Field*

It says the unsayable.
Gives voice to the voiceless.
It's a lifetime's work –
Handiwork, whole body work.

It gives form to chaos.
It reflects the present moment,
Changes the past
And creates the future.

It can exist forever
Or completely disappear.
It is what it is.
It can always be changed.

It's where the impossible
Becomes the possible.
It takes us out of ourselves
And into ourselves.

It is where we live our unlived lives,
Where we can surprise ourselves.
It is fire.
Only we can write our writing.

Map of the Book

Type of writing	Chapter	
Acrostics	Chapter 1	(Larry Butler)
Accompanying other art forms	Chapter 3	(Gillie Bolton)
	Chapter 6	(Kate Evans)
	Chapter 8	(River Wolton)
	Chapter 9	(Jo Monks)
AlphaPoems	Chapter 1	(Kathleen Adams)
Autobiography	Chapter 9	(Angie Butler)
Collaborative writing	Chapter 1	(Kathleen Adams, Cheryl Moskowitz, Kate D'Lima)
Diary	Chapter 8	(Irmeli Laitinen)
	Chapter 10	(Briony Goffin)
Form	Chapter 5	(Gillie Bolton, Kate Thompson, Robert Hamberger, Cheryl Moskowitz)
Freewriting	Chapter 6	(Dominique De-Light)
	Chapter 8	(Steven Weir, River Wolton)
	Chapter 9	(John Hilsdon)
	Chapter 10	(Briony Goffin)
Outside	Chapter 1	(Cheryl Moskowitz)
	Chapter 2	(Judy Clinton, Carrie Gorney)
Scribing for others	Chapter 1	(Kate D'Lima)
	Chapter 10	(Judy Clinton, Carrie Gorney)
Storytelling	Chapter 1	(Kate D'Lima)
	Chapter 10	(Carrie Gorney)
Unsent letters	Chapter 6	(Kathleen Adams)
	Chapter 10	(Kate Thompson)
Visualisation	Chapter 2	(Susan Kersley, Myra Schneider)
With talking	Chapter 6	(Kathleen Adams)
	Chapter 8	(River Wolton)
	Chapter 9	(Jo Monks)
	Chapter 10	(Kate Thompson)

Client group	Chapter	
Cancer patients	Chapter 4	(Fiona Hamilton)
	Chapter 6	(Fiona Hamilton)
	Chapter 9	(Gillie Bolton)
Children/young people	Chapter 4	(Roselle Angwin)
	Chapter 9	(Angie Butler, Gillie Bolton)
	Chapter 10	(Carrie Gorney)
Community carers/ social services	Chapter 3	(Glynis Charlton)
Counselling/ psychotherapy clients	Chapter 3	(Angela Stoner)
	Chapter 6	(Kathleen Adams)
	Chapter 7	(Geri Giebel Chavis, Monica Suswin)
	Chapter 10	(Kate Thompson, Carrie Gorney)
Doctors	Chapter 2	(Susan Kersley)
Elderly	Chapter 3	(Fiona Hamilton)
	Chapter 9	(Angie Butler)
Homeless	Chapter 6	(Dominique De-Light)
Hospital patients	Chapter 3	(Fiona Hamilton)
	Chapter 4	(Patricia L. Grant)
	Chapter 9	(Rose Flint)
Lifelong learning	Chapter 1	(Victoria Field)
	Chapter 3	(Geraldine Green)
	Chapter 4	(Miriam Halahmy)
	Chapter 5	(Kate Thompson)
	Chapter 7	(Alison Clayburn, Reinekke Lengelle)
	Chapter 8	(Annette Ecuyeré Lee)
	Chapter 9	(John Hilsdon)
Mental health	Chapter 1	(Kathleen Adams)
	Chapter 6	(Dominique De-Light, Kate Evans)
	Chapter 8	(Irmeli Laitinen, River Wolton)
	Chapter 9	(Gillie Bolton)
Peer training	Chapter 1	(Zeeba Ansara, Angie Butler)
	Chapter 3	(Gillie Bolton, Helen Boden)
	Chapter 6	(Jeannie Wright)
	Chapter 8	(Steven Wier)
	Chapter 9	(Jo Monks)

Themes	Chapter	
Childhood/birth	Chapter 6	(Maria Antoniou)
	Chapter 10	(Christine Bousfield)
Colour	Chapter 3	(Gillie Bolton)
Illness	Chapter 10	(Judy Clinton, Christine Bousfield)
Life aims and goals	Chapter 6	(Jeannie Wright)
	Chapter 8	(Steven Weir, River Wolton, Annette Ecuyeré Lee, Irmeli Laitinen)
Place	Chapter 3	(Geraldine Green, Helen Boden)
	Chapter 9	(Rose Flint)
Redrafting/ self-criticism	Chapter 9	(John Hilsdon)
Relationships	Chapter 6	(Kathleen Adams)
	Chapter 10	(Christine Bousfield, Kate Thompson)
Reminiscence	Chapter 8	(Irmmeli Laitinen)
	Chapter 9	(Angie Butler)

Classic Exercises

Useful Resources

These organisations will be of interest to those working with therapeutic writing. Most websites offer links to other relevant groups and organisations.

Apples and Snakes
England's leading organisers of performance poetry – stretching the boundaries of poetry in performance and education.

www.applesandsnakes.org

Federation of Worker Writers and Community Publishers
Umbrella organisation of over 80 writers' groups, and community-based publishers and organisations, who use words to enable people to have a voice.

www.thefwwcp.org.uk

Lapidus (the Association for Literary Arts in Personal Development)
Lapidus is the UK's organisation for anyone interested in the use of creative words to promote health and well-being.

Lapidus, BM Lapidus, London WC1N 3XX, UK
Tel: 0845 602 2215
www.lapidus.org.uk
info@lapidus.org.uk

literaturetraining
Offers information on training or professional development for members of a consortium of literature organisations in the UK. This consortium includes Lapidus; the other members are listed below with their websites.

literaturetraining, PO BOX 23595, Edinburgh EH6 7YX, UK
Tel: 0131 476 4039
www.literaturetraining.com
info@literaturetraining.com

NAPT (the National Association for Poetry Therapy)
Based in the US and offers training programmes in poetry/bibliotherapy.

Sheila Dietz, NAPT Administrator, 525 SW 5th Street, Suite A, Des Moines, Iowa 50309-4501, USA

Tel, toll-free: 1 866 844 NAPT; local: 515 282 8192; fax: 515 282 9117
www.poetrytherapy.org
info@poetrytherapy.org

NNAH (National Network for the Arts in Health)

An advocate for the arts in the health field, bringing together the arts and health communities and disseminating a wealth of information, resources and products.

National Network for the Arts in Health, The Menier Chocolate Factory, 51 Southwark Street, London SE1 1RU, UK
Tel: 0870 143 4555
info@nnah.org.uk

Scottish Book Trust

Scotland's national agency for reading and writing.

www.scottishbooktrust.com

Survivors' Poetry

Promotes the poetry of survivors of mental distress.

www.survivorspoetry.com

The National Association for Literature Development

The professional body for all involved in developing writers, readers and literature audiences.

www.nald.org

The National Association of Writers in Education (lead partner)

The one organisation supporting writers and writing of all genres in all educational settings throughout the UK.

www.nawe.co.uk

writernet

Provides dramatic writers with the tools to build better careers and redefine the culture in which they work.

www.writernet.org.uk

Websites of organisations and individuals working in the area of therapeutic writing:

www.gilliebolton.com
www.victoriafield.co.uk
www.journaltherapy.com
www.journaltherapy.co.uk
www.poeticmedicine.com
www.wordsworthcenter.com

References

Adams, K. (1990) *Journal to the Self.* New York: Warner Books.

Armitage, S. (1993) 'Mother, any distance greater than a single span' in *Book of Matches.* London: Faber & Faber.

Bolton, G. (1999) *The Therapeutic Potential of Creative Writing: Writing Myself.* London: Jessica Kingsley Publishers.

Bolton, G. (2000) 'On Becoming our Own Shaman: Creative Writing as Therapy.' *Context: The Magazine for Family Therapy and Systemic Practice,* 47, pp.18–20.

Bolton, G. (2001) 'Open the Box: Writing a Therapeutic Space' in P. Milner (ed.) *BAC Counselling Reader, Volume 2.* London: Sage Publications, pp. 106–12.

Bolton, G. (2003) 'Around the Slices of Herself' in K. Etherington (ed.) *Trauma, the Body and Transformation: A Narrative Enquiry.* London: Jessica Kingsley Publishers.

Bolton, G. (2005) 'Medicine and Literature: Writing and Reading.' *Journal of Evaluation in Clinical Practice,* 1 (2), 171–9.

Bolton, G. and Stoner, A. (2004) 'Follow the Mind's Wings: Therapeutic Writing.' *Context: The Magazine for Family Therapy and Systemic Practice,* 75, October, 22–4.

Bolton, G., Howlett, S., Lago, C. and Wright, J. (2002) *Writing Cures: An Introductory Handbook of Writing in Counselling and Psychotherapy.* London: Brunner-Routledge.

Brande, D. (1996) *Becoming a Writer.* London: Pan.

Burgess, A. (1986) *The Piano Players.* London: Hutchinson.

Cameron, J. (1994) *The Artist's Way: A Course in Discovering and Recovering Your Creative Self.* London: Pan.

Clayburn, A. (2002) 'This Black Cloud Has a Life of Its Own.' *Mslexia 13,* Spring/Summer.

Duff, K. (1993) *The Alchemy of Illness.* New York: Random House.

Elbow, P. (1998) *Writing Without Teachers.* New York: Oxford University Press.

Field, V. (2004a) 'A Sort-of Sonnet' in D. Hart (ed.) *Freedom Rules: New Forms for the Making of Poems.* Birmingham: Flarestack.

Field, V. (2004b) 'Words' in *Olga's Dreams.* Truro, Cornwall: fal publications.

Flint, R. (2000) 'Fragile Space: Therapeutic Relationship and the Word' in F. Sampson (ed.) *Writing in Health and Social Care.* London: Jessica Kingsley Publishers.

Ford, D. (1998) *Dark Side of the Light Chasers: Reclaiming Your Power, Creativity, Brilliance, and Dreams.* New York: Riverhead Books.

Fox, J. (1997) *Poetic Medicine: The Healing Art of Poem Making.* New York: Penguin Putnam.

Freud, S. [1919] (1985) 'The Uncanny' in *Art and Literature Pelican Freud Library, Volume 14.* London and New York: Penguin. (First published in 1919).

Frost, R. (1935) Address, 17 May. Milton Academy, MA.

Frost, R. (1971) 'Come In' in I. Hamilton (ed.) *Selected Poems.* London: Penguin.

Glaister, L. (2004) *As Far As You Can Go.* London: Bloomsbury.

Glouberman, D. (1995) *Life Choices, Life Changes: Develop Your Personal Vision with Imagework*. London: Thorsons.

Goldberg, N. (1986) *Writing Down The Bones*. Boston, MA: Shambhala.

Goldberg, N. (1991) *Wild Mind*. New York: Random House.

Greenlaw, L. (1993) 'From Scattered Blue' in *Night Photograph*. London: Faber and Faber.

Guillen, N. (2004) *The Great Zoo and Other Poems*, translated and edited by R. Marquez. London: Mango Publishing.

Hamberger, R. (1997) *Warpaint Angel*. Nottingham: Blackwater Press c/o Five Leaves Publications.

Hartley Williams, J. and Sweeney, M. (1997) *Teach Yourself Writing Poetry*. London: Hodder Headline.

Hayes, K. (1999) *Bridge of Shadows*. London: Black Swan.

Hayes, K. (2005) *The Writing Game*. Bath: Globe IQ.

Heaney, S. (1984) 'A Kite for Michael and Christopher' in *Station Island*. London: Faber & Faber.

Higher Awareness (2001) 'What is Your Life Purpose?' *Inner Journey Weekly Workout, 5–50*. Online at www.higherawareness.com. Site visited 11 December.

Hilsdon, J. (2004) 'After the Session – Notemaking in Counselling and Psychotherapy' in G. Bolton, S. Howlett, C. Lago and J. Wright (eds) *Writing Cures*. London: Brunner-Routledge.

Hopkins, G.M. (1953) *Poems and Prose of Gerard Manley Hopkins*. London: Penguin.

Hudson, F.M. (1999) *Revised Edition Mastering the Art of Self-Renewal: Adulthood as Continual Revitalization*. New York: MJF Books (Fine Communications).

Hynes, A.A.M. and Hynes Berry, M. (1994) *Biblio/Poetry Therapy: The Interactive Process: A Handbook*. St. Cloud, MN: North Star Press.

Jones, L.B. (1996) *The Path: Creating Your Mission Statement for Work and for Life*. New York: Hyperion Press.

King, S.K. (1990) *Urban Shaman*. New York: Fireside.

Knights, B. (1995) *The Listening Reader – Fiction and Poetry for Counsellors and Psychotherapists*. London: Jessica Kingsley Publishers.

Koch, K. (1977) *I Never Told Anybody – Teaching Poetry Writing in a Nursing Home*. New York: Random House.

Koch, K. (1996) *The Art of Poetry – Poems, Parodies, Interviews, Essays and Other Work*. Ann Arbor, MI: University of Michigan.

Leider, R. J. (1994) *Life Skills: Taking Charge of Your Personal and Professional Growth*. San Diego, CA: Pfeiffer & Company.

Lepore, S.J. and Smyth, J.M. (2002) *The Writing Cure*. Washington, DC: American Psychological Association.

Maguire, S. (1997) 'No. 3 Greenhouse, 7.30a.m.' in *The Invisible Mender*. London: Cape.

March, C. (ed.) (1998) *Knowing ME: Women Speak about Myalgic Encephalomyelitis and Chronic Fatigue Syndrome*. London: The Women's Press.

Martin, R.B. (1991) *Gerard Manley Hopkins: A Very Private Life*. London: Flamingo/ Harper Collins.

Matthews, P. (1994) *Sing Me the Creation – A Sourcebook for Poets and Teachers, and for all who wish to Develop the Life of the Imagination*. Stroud: Hawthorn Press.

Mazza, N. (1993) *Poetry Therapy: Theory and Practice*. London: Brunner-Routledge.

McEwen, C. and Statman, M. (2000) *The Alphabet of the Trees*. New York: Teachers and Writers Collaborative.

McGough, R. (1999) *The Way Things Are*. London: Viking (Penguin).

McKendrick, J. (2003) 'Apotheosis' in *Ink Stone*. London: Faber & Faber.

Michaels, A. (1996) *Fugitive Pieces*. London: Bloomsbury.

Mindell, A. (1993) *The Shaman's Body*. San Francisco: Harper Collins.

Neruda, P. (1972) 'We are Many' in *Collected Poems*, translated by Alastair Reid. London: Cape Goliard Press.

ni Dhomhnaill, N. (2002) 'The Language Issue' translated by Paul Muldoon in Neil Astley (ed.) *Staying Alive*. Newcastle: Bloodaxe.

Olds, S. (1987) *The Gold Cell*. New York: Alfred Knopf.

Paterson, D. (1999) *101 Sonnets from Shakespeare to Heaney*. Edited with an introduction by Don Paterson. London: Faber & Faber.

Pennebaker, J.W. (1997) *Opening Up: The Healing Power of Expressing Emotions*. New York: Guildford.

Perls, F.S. (1971) *Gestalt Therapy Verbatim*. London: Bantam.

Plath, S. (1998) 'The Arrival of the Bee Box' in S. Armitage and R. Crawford (eds) *The Penguin Book of Poetry from Britain and Ireland Since 1945*. London: Viking.

Robbins, A. (2001) *Unlimited Power*. London: Pocket Books.

Rowan, A. and Harper, E. (1999) 'Group Subversion as Subjective Necessity – Towards a Lacanian Orientation to Psychoanalysis in Group Settings' in C. Oakley (ed.) *What is a Group?* London: Rebus Press.

Rumi (1995) 'The Guest House' in *The Essential Rumi* translated by Coleman Barks with J. Moyne. San Francisco, CA: Harper Collins.

Sansom, P. (1994) *Writing Poems*. Newcastle: Bloodaxe.

Schneider, M. (2003) *Writing My Way Through Cancer*. London: Jessica Kingsley Publishers.

Schneider, M. and Killick, J. (1998) *Writing for Self-Discovery*. Shaftesbury: Element.

St Vincent Millay, E. (1988) *Collected Sonnets*. New York: Harper and Row.

Stevens, W. (1982) 'Thirteen Ways of Looking at a Blackbird' in S. Heaney and T. Hughes (ed.) *The Rattle Bag*. London: Faber and Faber.

Stryk, L. (tr.) (1985) *On Love and Barley: Haiku of Basho*. London: Penguin.

Thomas, D. (1998) 'Do Not Go Gentle Into that Good Night', in M. Hart and J. Loader (eds) *Generations: Poems between Fathers, Mothers, Daughters, Sons*. London: Penguin.

Woolf, V. (1978) *Moments of Being*. Gainesville: Triad Books.

Wordsworth, W. (1975) 'Composed upon Westminster Bridge' in W. Davies (ed.) *Selected Poems*. London: J.M. Dent.

Wright, J. (2005) 'Writing Therapy in Brief Workplace Counselling.' *Counselling and Psychotherapy Research Journal*, 5 (2), pp.111–19.

Yalom, I. (1985) *The Theory and Practice of Group Psychotherapy*, Third Edition. New York: Basic Books.

Contributors

Kathleen Adams, licensed psychotherapist and registered poetry/journal therapist from Denver, Colorado, USA, is the author of six books on therapeutic writing, including the bestselling *Journal to the Self* (Warner Books, 1990). Kathleen is the founder-director of the Center for Journal Therapy (www.journaltherapy.com) and is considered one of the leading theorists in the interface between journal writing and healing.

Roselle Angwin is a poet, author and director of the Fire in the Head creative and reflective writing programme. Her work hinges on the connections between self and self/other, self and place, and creativity and well-being. Recent books are *Writing the Bright Moment* and *Looking For Icarus.*

Zeeba Ansari is a poet and poetry tutor. She works in partnership with Cornwall Library and Adult Education Services, facilitating poetry groups for adults. Zeeba also runs The Poetry Practice, mentoring individual poets and running courses and workshops. The exploration and development of individual responses to creativity, and their broader implications, are key elements in her approach.

Maria Antoniou writes creative autobiography. Her PhD thesis (submitted in 2002 at the University of Manchester) used a variety of writing forms to explore aspects of her embodied identity. She teaches creative writing to academic researchers and is starting to facilitate workshops using writing for personal development.

Helen Boden is a freelance facilitator, editor and writer based in Edinburgh. She runs courses and workshops on writing for well-being and writing and walking, and has recently produced an anthology of her clients' work, *Wild On Her Blue Days.* Relentlessly fascinated by the dynamism of language, she is also inspired by landscape, music and good food.

Gillie Bolton has been working and writing in the field of therapeutic creative writing for 30 years, having discovered it worked for her own private therapy. Having veered from social anthropology to teaching creative writing, she found herself in medicine and health by chance and has never looked back. She is author of *Reflective Practice Writing for Professional Development*, Second Edition (Sage, 2005), and *The Therapeutic Potential of Creative Writing: Writing Myself* (Jessica Kingsley Publishers, 1999); co-editor of *Writing Cures: An Introductory Handbook of Writing in Counselling and Psychotherapy* (Brunner-Routledge, 2004); literature and medicine editor to the *Journal* *of Medical Humanities* (BMJ); health and arts editor to *Progress in Palliative Care*; poetry editor to *Spirituality and Health International*; associate editor to *The Journal of Poetry Therapy*; founder member of the Council of the UK Association for Medical Humanities; and a poet.

Christine Bousfield is a lecturer and poet who runs poetry therapy workshops. She has poems in magazines such as *The North, Orbis* and *Dream Catcher*, on BBC's *The Weekend Poem*, and on CD with Nightdiver Poetry Jazz who regularly perform live. She is currently working on a collection, *Tense Formations*.

Angie Butler is a retired teacher and a self-published author of five children's books. She has been involved in hospital radio, where she read stories with children and parents on the children's ward. A supply teacher, she runs art and language workshops, and is an adult education tutor and member of Lapidus.

Larry Butler is a Tai-Chi teacher, creative writing facilitator and co-founder of the Poetry Healing Project from which he developed Survivors' Poetry Scotland. He is convenor of Lapidus Scotland. He recently completed a feasibility study for the Greater Glasgow Health Board on the idea of 'Arts on Prescription'.

Glynis Charlton started writing when her marriage ended and has since developed a whole new life. Having ditched the day job, she now works freelance, evaluating arts projects and running creative writing workshops. She particularly engages with those experiencing a tough time, seeing her role as facilitator who enables people to be introspective.

Geri Giebel Chavis is a licensed psychologist, certified poetry therapist and mentor-supervisor; she counsels groups, individuals, couples and families in Minnesota, USA. As professor at the College of St Catherine in St Paul, Minnesota, Geri teaches literature and biblio/poetry courses and leads poetry therapy workshops in the USA, Britain and Ireland. Geri is executive board member of the National Association for Poetry Therapy and honorary president of the Irish Poetry Therapy Network.

Alison Clayburn is writer of poetry and short prose. She lives in London, by the Thames. After a long career as a community worker she became an adult educator, specialising in creative writing for personal development. She describes herself as a 'writing groupie' who gains much from workshops and writers' networks.

Judy Clinton facilitates writing workshops for personal and spiritual development in retreat centres and elsewhere. She is a trained teacher and published writer, and has worked in the social care and counselling fields in various capacities. Her work combines all her personal and professional experiences with her Quaker outlook on life.

Dominique De-Light was initially a travel writer and Rough Guide author. She gained an MA in creative writing from the University of East Anglia in 2001. She ran the Brighton Big Issue writing group for four years, is the writer in residence for a day centre for homeless adults and is a Lapidus mentor.

Kate D'Lima is Lecturer in Performing Arts, Writing and Literature in the Department of Adult Continuing Education, Swansea University. She has an MA in the teaching and practice of creative writing and is researching creative writing in health settings for her PhD. She is also an award-winning writer of fiction.

Kate Evans used to write mainly for publication until a devastating bout of depression, then she began to write madly, personally and eventually therapeutically. Currently writing poetry and a book, she teaches on the University of Hull's Certificate in Creative Writing and facilitates groups in community and mental health settings.

Victoria Field was born in London in 1963. Her first degree is in psychology in which she lectured for three years before joining the British Council and serving in Turkey, Russia and Pakistan. She has a lifelong love of language and languages and on return to the UK was appointed Director of Survivors' Poetry. She subsequently moved to Cornwall where she combined her interests in literature and psychology by training and working as a poetry therapist in NHS, education and other settings. She has a long association with Lapidus, including two spells as Chair, and is on the board of the NAPT Foundation and the editorial board of *The Journal of Poetry Therapy*. She is a prize-winning writer of poetry, fiction and drama. Her first collection of poetry is *Olga's Dreams* (fal publications, 2004) and her second professionally produced play, *Glass Heart*, commissioned by Hall for Cornwall, toured in 2006.

Rose Flint is both poet and art therapist. As lead writer for the Kingfisher Project, Salisbury, she runs groups in varied community and hospital settings. She works primarily as a poet, trusting poetry and its relationship to the inner world to deliver a therapeutic value. Her latest collection is *Nekyia* (Stride; 2003).

Briony Goffin gained a BSc in psychology and an MA in the teaching and practice of creative writing at Cardiff University. She now facilitates creative writing groups for adults with mental health problems in Cardiff. She also teaches her independent courses on creative and autobiographical writing in Somerset.

Linda Goodwin works as a freelance practitioner using the potential of creative writing to enhance the well-being of her students. Through the use of experimental writing stimuli she helps individuals draw on their creative core; recognising their creative capabilities through supportive workshop sessions.

Carry Gorney works as a systemic psychotherapist in the NHS, with families and children. She says, 'We listen to and tell stories. Achievements and dilemmas of the present reflect stories of the past. We talk, write and draw to create the hopes and dreams of an illuminated future.'

Patricia L. Grant holds a Masters of Literature, a Masters in social work, and a doctorate in education. She knows from personal experience that writing poetry heals even a seared-scarred soul. She believes that all people are creative, that each person has an unique voice expressed through their poetry, which enhances all of us.

Geraldine Green's first collection *The Skin* was published in 2002 by Flarestack. She graduated in 2005 with an MA (distinction) in creative writing, Lancaster University; lives in Cumbria; and runs writing workshops and is a tutor for Continuing Education. Currently working on her third collection, her second, *Passio*, was published in 2006 by Flarestack.

Miriam Halahmy is a freelance writer and workshop facilitator. She was Chair of Lapidus 2003–5 and is poetry editor of the *Lapidus Quarterly*. Miriam has published two poetry collections, a novel and resources for schools. She has facilitated workshops with the homeless and ex-offenders. Miriam is currently completing a book for children with cancer, sponsored by CancerBacup.

Robert Hamberger's poetry has appeared in numerous magazines, including the *Observer, New Statesman*, the *Spectator, Poetry Review* and *Gay Times*. He has been awarded a Hawthornden Fellowship and shortlisted for a Forward Prize. He has published two collections: *Warpaint Angel* (Blackwater Press, 1997) and *The Smug Bridegroom* (Five Leaves, 2002).

Fiona Hamilton set up Writing in Healthcare in 2002 to provide creative writing sessions in health settings including the Children's Hospital in Bristol, where she is writer in residence, and the Bristol Cancer Help Centre, which incorporated her courses into its regular programme in 2005. She won the Belmont Poetry Prize in 2005.

David Hart, born in Aberystwyth, formerly Birmingham University chaplain, theatre critic and arts administrator, is now a freelance poet, has been writer-in-residence in psychiatric and general hospitals and at Worcester Cathedral, and lectures part-time at Warwick and Birmingham universities. Birmingham Poet Laureate 1997–8, he won First and Second in the National Poetry Competition.

Graham Hartill has lived mostly in Wales for the last 30 years. Poet and workshop facilitator, he has taught and presented his work in numerous universities and institutions throughout the UK and the USA and was a co-founder of Lapidus. His selected poems, *Cennau's Bell*, were published in 2005 by the Collective Press.

John Hilsdon is a lecturer at the University of Plymouth, where he teaches and writes in the field of learning development. He also works as a counsellor for the Macmillan Centre at Derriford Hospital. John is a National Teaching Fellow and founder of the Learning Development in Higher Education Network (LDHEN).

Susan Kersley is a life coach, neurolinguistic programming practitioner and retired doctor. She works with stressed and overworked doctors who want a life. She is the author of *Prescription for Change* (2005) and the *ABC of Change for Doctors* (2006), both published by Radcliffe.

Irmeli Laitinen was born in Finland where she has trained as a psychoanalytic psychotherapist. She is a co-founder of the Women's Therapy Centre in Helsinki and she has been working in the Women's Therapy Centre in London. Currently she works as a psychoanalytic psychotherapist at the NHS Eating Disorders Clinic in Truro, Cornwall.

Annette Ecuyeré Lee lives in west Wales where she supports authors, businesses and students with their writing on a daily basis, as well as teaching creative writing workshops and running an annual Festival of Writing. She has a PGDip in creative writing and personal development and is completing an MA in entrepreneurial management.

Reinekke Lengelle is a professor at Athabasca University in Canada. 'Writing the Self' is the online graduate course she designed and teaches for AU. Reinekke was also writer-in-residence with the Artist-on-the-Wards at the University of Alberta hospital for three years. She is a poet, playwright, self-help author and publisher – www.blacktulippress.com.

Debbie McCulliss, a nurse for 30 years, became passionate about writing six years ago when she began to research her family history and write her autobiography. Today she is also passionate about inspiring others to write. She is a facilitator of women's writing groups, a poetry/journal therapist- in-training and a student of creative writing.

Dominic McLoughlin has run creative writing workshops in many healthcare settings and teaches on the MA in creative writing and personal development at the University of Sussex. His poems appear in *Entering the Tapestry* (Enitharmon, 2003) and online at www.poetrypf.co.uk. Dominic's chapter on poetry writing in a hospice appeared in *Creative Writing in Health and Social Care* (Jessica Kingsley Publishers, 2004).

Jo Monks is a creative arts facilitator using storytelling, drama and creative writing to enable people to express themselves and tell their own personal stories through a multi-arts approach. She runs group and one-to-one healing arts sessions in East Sussex and works in collaboration with healer, holistic therapist and life coach Jabeen.

Cheryl Moskowitz is a poet, playwright and novelist. Trained in psychodynamic counselling, she tutors on the MA in creative writing and personal development at the University of Sussex and works extensively as a writer in schools and in the community. Her poems are in several anthologies. Her autobiographical novel, *Wyoming Trail*, was published by Granta in 1998.

Sherry Reiter, PhD, is a clinical social worker who is also registered as a poetry and drama therapist. She is the director of The Creative Righting Center in New York City, where she offers a regional and distance poetry therapy training programme. Sherry is recipient of the 2005 NAPT Art Lerner Pioneer Award for her visionary work in the field. She divides her work between university teaching, writing and private practice.

Leone Ridsdale works as a neurologist with responsibility for organising clinical teaching at Guy's, King's and St Thomas's Hospitals, London. Her interests include developing community services for people with fatigue, headache and epilepsy. She has adopted children who are now teenagers, and sees writing as a form of personal therapy.

Myra Schneider is a poet and a creative writing tutor. Her most recent poetry collection is *Multiplying the Moon* (Enitharmon, 2004). She is very interested in personal and therapeutic writing and her book *Writing My Way Through Cancer* (Jessica Kingsley Publishers, 2003) is a fleshed-out journal with poems and writing suggestions. She also co-wrote, with John Killick, *Writing for Self-Discovery* (Element, 1998).

Angela Stoner is a former English and drama teacher who now facilitates a number of personal development and writing groups, in a variety of settings. She doesn't see herself as a tutor or therapist, but as someone who helps people to reconnect, through writing, with their own inner sources of healing and strength.

Monica Suswin is a writer and workshop facilitator. She has a background in psychotherapy and journalism (BBC Radio Four), and an MA in creative writing from the University of Sussex (2002). A growing awareness of therapeutic writing – for herself and for others – has become a home-coming weaving the different strands of her life together.

Kate Thompson read English at Cambridge and after teaching for some years retrained as a counsellor. She has worked in private practice and the NHS. When living in Boulder, Colorado, she discovered the Center for Journal Therapy where her two passions, literature and therapy, came together. She uses journal writing as a therapeutic tool with clients and supervisees, both online and face-to-face, and trains professionals in its use. She has published widely on the subject and is Vice-Chair of Lapidus. She lives in the Derbyshire Dales. Reading and writing and walking in the hills are how she makes sense of the world.

Jane Tozer has an English degree (Cambridge: New Hall) and was Chair of Falmouth Poetry Group 1999–2005. Grant-aided by Arts Council England, South West, her version of the twelfth-century Lais of Marie de France has won two translation prizes. The Arvon Foundation and Taliesin Trust restored her confidence; her artist husband inspires her every day.

Elaine Trevitt trained as an osteopath and has 20 years' experience working with the body/mind/spirit interface. She works intuitively and eclectically but remains deeply grounded in anatomy and physiology. She believes that writing can encourage a person towards optimal health, being one expression of the 'inner physician'.

Steven Weir is a writer and life coach. His love for mapping the inner landscape has led him to develop tools that enable us to tap into our most valuable resources. His workshop in this book facilitated such a process, where each participant became their own teacher.

Claire Williamson is a writer with an MA in literary studies and a certificate in counselling. Her narrative book of poems *Ride On* was released with Arts Council backing in 2005. Claire has worked in a variety of community settings including schools, prisons and addiction and health-care settings.

River Wolton is a poet and playwright based in Sheffield. She trained in social work, practised as a psychotherapist for ten years and now facilitates creative and reflective writing in a wide range of community projects, schools and adult education.

Jeannie Wright has been writing what she cannot say since an early age. Accredited with the British Association for Counselling and Psychotherapy since 1993 and interested in innovative practice, her research and recent publications reflect this interest, focusing on the therapeutic potential of creative writing and writing as a vehicle for reflective practice and personal and professional development.

Subject Index

Author
Index

Lightning Source UK Ltd.
Milton Keynes UK
UKOW03f0031090813

215082UK00001B/2/P